Praise for *Intact: Unta_____ _____ ____ Depression, Addiction, and Trauma*

"At times laugh-out-loud, at times cry-out-loud, Kildare takes you on her journey toward overcoming trauma and reconnecting with self and details her hard-won battle learning how to manage addiction and bipolar depression."
—Bobbie Oliver stand-up comic, comedy coach, and author of *The Tao of Comedy: Embrace the Pause*

"Kildare shares her gripping story, research, and insights into the intricacies of bipolar depression and how overcoming childhood trauma became the critical first step toward learning how to manage bipolar and addiction."
—Sheila Hamilton, Five-time Emmy Award-winning journalist and author of "All the Things We Never Knew"

"Through her raw, honest, and vulnerable storytelling, Kildare shares her lifelong journey of overcoming trauma, co-occurring bipolar and addiction disorders as well as demonstrating the power of perseverance and self-discovery found in recovery."
—Karl Shallowhorn, President of Shallowhorn Consulting, LLC and author of *Working on Wellness: A Practical Guide to Mental Health*

"Compelling. As well as sharing her journey from the depths of psychosis to leading a healthy, productive life, Kildare spells out the many tools she uses to manage the symptoms of bipolar depression."
—Joanne Doan, Publisher mental health magazines *bp Magazine* and *Esperanza*

Intact

ALSO BY SASHA KILDARE

Dream Walking

Intact

Untangle the Web of Bipolar Depression, Addiction, and Trauma

A Memoir and Information Guide

Sasha Kildare

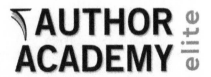

Printed in the United States of America

Published by Author Academy Elite
PO Box 43, Powell, OH 43065
www.AuthorAcademyElite.com

Library of Congress Cataloging: 2020926053
Softcover: 978-1-64746-663-3
Hardcover: 978-1-64746-664-0
E-book: 978-1-64746-665-7

Available in paperback, hardback, e-book, and audiobook

Any Internet addresses (websites, blogs, etc.) and telephone numbers printed in this book are offered as a resource. They are not intended in any way to be or imply an endorsement by Author Academy Elite, nor does Author Academy Elite vouch for the content of these sites and numbers for the life of this book.

The memoir chapters of this book depict actual events in the life of the author as truthfully as recollection permits and/or can be verified by research. Some names have been changed to respect the privacy of those individuals.

Book design by Jet Launch.
Cover design by Debbie O'Byrne.

To those who are tasked with untangling their webs.

To those wounded healers who advance the healing of others struggling with mental health.

To those who make advances in the treatment of mental health possible.

"What mental health needs is more sunlight, more candor, and more unashamed conversation." – Glenn Close

Table of Contents

Part Two: Chaos

Part Three: Awareness

Part Four: Awakening

Part Five: Insight

Foreword

For the past seven years, Sasha Kildare has been one of NAMI Greater Los Angeles County's *In Our Own Voice* presenters who share the story of their lives with community groups of What Happened, What Helps, and What's Next related to coping with their mental health challenge.

She shares her story, because of her gratitude for her living well today and her desire to fight the stigma that stands in the way of more widespread, effective treatments for people living with mental health conditions. *Intact: Untangling the Web of Bipolar Depression, Addiction, and Trauma* is a memoir as well as an information guide and presents brief interviews and easy-to-read summaries of recent research concerning treatment.

In it, she starkly depicts young adult summers during which she was hospitalized numerous times and her judgment was so impaired in the throes of mania that she placed herself in numerous life-threatening situations. Her ability to reclaim her life and sustain long-term recovery has been due to many factors, not the least of which is the community and support provided by organizations including NAMI. In addition to working full-time and raising two children, for the past 10 years, Sasha contributes mental health feature articles to *Esperanza* and *bp Magazine*.

Brain disorders are complex, and generally require multi-pronged treatment including lifestyle accommodations. Sasha's journey necessitated coming to terms with addiction and childhood trauma and trying out various other coping strategies. You'll be as fascinated, educated, and inspired by her perseverance as I am once you finish this book.

Brittney Weissman
CEO, NAMI Greater Los Angeles County

Acknowledgments

I would like to thank Bellevue Hospital for providing me with the wraparound treatment that changed the course of my life. Bellevue's outpatient program led me to "Sarah," a gifted therapist, who helped me release my buried pain and gave me tools to disarm its triggers.

Patrick and Laura—my fiercely independent, responsible, and kind children—thank you for the joy you bring me. I am deeply grateful for the education Long Beach Unified School District has provided you and that you both embrace athletic and academic challenges.

A thousand thank yous to my one and only sibling for tracking us down and becoming Patrick and Laura's adventurous "Uncle Mike."

Two long-time friends consistently spark my creativity. My writing buddy since college, Angela Haugh, shares her originality and inspiration with me. Katrina Hagen-Swanson inspires me with her honesty, integrity, sense of humor, and thoughtful gifts. Included in one gift bag was a refrigerator magnet that quotes the Dalai Lama, "My religion is very simple. My religion is kindness."

Within the last few years, two childhood friends tracked me down. Tanya and Carla take me back to that carefree time in my childhood when lawns were for learning to turn cartwheels and trees were for climbing.

The Igniting Souls Tribe, including author/writing coach extraordinaire Daphne Smith, have nourished my soul, my storytelling, and my confidence.

I'm grateful for the magnificent community NAMI has created and for their undaunting effort to reduce stigma by raising public awareness, creating opportunities, and providing education and programs that support individuals and families affected by mental illness.

INTRODUCTION

The Web

What would happen if an illness reprogrammed your brain? Scrambled your character traits? Prudent reset to promiscuous. Cautious to reckless. Who would you become? Would you be able to take care of yourself?

My young adult experiences still seem unbelievable to me—near-anonymous sex facilitated by drugs and several psychotic, manic, breaks from reality. These breaks drew out my doppelganger and earned me seven trips to the psych ward.

My journey was surreal, psychedelic, terrifying, and, at times, exhilarating and erotic.

My psychotic episodes seem like nightmares, except they really happened. Impulsivity ruled me, and I lost the ability to take care of myself. The worst part is that I remember everything.

Whatever disassociation I used to survive child abuse, some strength in my spirit survived until I ended up in a psych ward at 18.

Whatever disassociation I used to survive child abuse, some strength in my spirit survived until I ended up in a psych ward at 18.

At 19, my binge eating disorder upgraded to binge drug addiction after being prescribed highly addictive "anxiety erasers," which led me to street drugs. My young adult journey through risky promiscuity, street life, and multiple hospitalizations was unnecessary because I had no idea what triggered my depression, post-traumatic stress, eating disorder, or mania.

Bipolar disorder, addiction, and the aftereffects of trauma can feed off of each other and become a tangled web of pain, despair, and isolation. Whether you are dealing with any of the three or all of the three, there is so much you can learn and do to become aware of how they influence each other, help manage them, and unlock patterns in the subconscious mind.

Through Q&A interviews, science-based tips written in a conversational voice, poetry, dark humor, and stories from my healing journey, I want to empower you by sharing with you what I wish I would have been taught at 18—many factors influence brain function. Circadian rhythms, processing challenges, addiction, lifestyle, nutrition, and other hormonal or health challenges are some of them.

Through changing your habits and examining your thought patterns, your brain can create beneficial new neural pathways and you can better connect to your spirit. For example, research shows that goal setting is a skill that you can acquire and so is gratitude.

It is not possible to manage bipolar disorder (also known as manic depression or bipolar or bipolar depression) if you have zero insight into the variety of factors that could influence it. The same holds true for addiction and for the aftereffects of trauma.

Whether you are in treatment, need treatment, a family member, a friend, a mental health professional, or simply curious, *Intact* gives insight into the mechanisms of all three conditions and explains the tools that can help combat them.

At the age of 26, I was lucky to receive wraparound treatment from New York City's Bellevue Hospital, my seventh, and last, hospitalization. It included follow-up outpatient care, health insurance, vocational counseling and training, supervised housing, and therapy, which revealed the negative voices, the flashbacks, and the buried pain. These resources sent me on a path toward healing my broken spirit, confronting my drug addiction, and learning how to manage bipolar disorder and identify its triggers. I was able to return to the workforce within eighteen months, and I regained a sense of hope that I could have a future beyond juggling minimum wage jobs. I was also lucky that my mood swings, even though severe, had been far apart enough that I knew what it was like to live symptom-free.

Eventually, I graduated from college and connected with a spiritual discipline that rejuvenated me and helped me adjust my thinking patterns and come to terms with trading addictions. My education gave me the skills necessary to research the factors that influence bipolar disorder and addiction and the strategies for managing these chronic conditions. This knowledge and access to healthcare enabled me to live a productive life including parenthood.

Integrative approach needed

In 2020, while suicide rates are declining in other parts of the world, including Japan, China, and most of Western Europe, they are rising in the US, particularly among young adults. The Substance Abuse and Mental Health Services Administration (SAMHSA) reports a tremendous unmet need for treatment for young adults grappling with addiction, mental health conditions, or both.

Although medication can be a critical part of managing a mental health condition, it's usually not the only tool needed.

If I parked myself in front of a grocery store and surveyed its customers by asking them, "Do you realize what you eat can influence depression," I would most likely be met with stares. Research shows nutrition can play a significant role in mental health as can so many other factors, but public awareness is not yet there.

Unpuzzling depression

Depressive episodes are part of bipolar disorder and can play a role in addiction. Even manic episodes can have mixed features of painful depression. My manic episodes always came out of episodes of depression that had escalated. Using a substance or thrill-seeking behavior made the pain go away. For a while.

Discovering the pieces of the puzzle that contribute to depression or that could trigger mania or substance abuse can go a long way toward minimizing episodes or nipping them in the bud. Also, sometimes the high sensitivity trait, sensory processing sensitivity, can influence depression.

Habits can help you

Habits are hard to change and so is culture. Proper nutrition, regular exercise, mindfulness, and goal-setting could all become part of the equation that helps to manage mental health conditions.

For me, the healthy habits, altered thinking patterns, and surrender eventually became mostly routine, and my battle became more like a chore.

So much goes into who we are and how we function or malfunction, such as neuroscience, compulsivity, spirituality, genetics, and trauma. Brains are our most complex organs, and our subconscious minds are linked to our souls.

What is mania?

Imagine a hyperactive two-year-old in an adult body. Brain scans reveal that the section of the brain responsible for judgment is all but shut down. Neurotransmitters and hormones run amok. Sex hormones are raging. The biochemistry of sex is remarkable. Sex can help you relax, and it can help you sleep. Sex provides a rush, but it can become a drug. Compulsive sex can ruin your life.

- Your energy is off the charts.

- You don't want to sleep.

- You can't stop thinking, imagining, doing.

- You're dreaming, but you're awake.

- Impaired judgment + hypersexuality + compulsivity = Disaster.

There is no blood test for bipolar. I hope that *Intact* helps demystify it, provides insight into its relationship with addiction and trauma, and offers tools that can help tame them.

A Note to the Reader

I began writing a novel in my early thirties right before having children. I had kept journals through the years, and the memories of childhood trauma, manic episodes, and hospitalizations I experienced during my young adult years were fresh.

After one year, I couldn't find my voice and began a memoir.

Many drafts later, I found an agent but ultimately decided against pursuing publication of the memoir, because I did not think it was in the best interests of my children at the time. Also, because of the Great Recession, I was afraid of workplace discrimination.

Fiction is my first love, and I turned the memoir into a novel, *Dream Walking* that I published in 2013. Also, in 2013, I began speaking for NAMI's In Our Own Voice program. NAMI's programs help to fill in the gaps and go a long way to helping fight stigma.

With one child in college and my second child in high school, in late 2018, I began writing a memoir again. What compelled me to write is the sadness I feel about the aspects of American culture that inadvertently contribute to brain disorders (another term for mental illness) and the lack of integrative treatments that would take into account addiction medicine, nutrition, processing challenges, and many more pieces of the puzzle that influence our most complex organ, the brain.

I ended up borrowing bits of *Dream Walking* that actually happened. Those chapters had gone through oodles of drafts, and I could not tell those pivotal events, such as my first and last hospitalizations, any better.

Terminology

Until the 1980 edition of the *Diagnostic and Statistical Manual of Mental Disorders* (DSM-3), bipolar disorder was called manic depression or manic-depressive illness. However, I prefer the term bipolar depression, because it reveals more. Bipolar disorder is also commonly referred to as bipolar. I mainly use the term bipolar disorder, but I use the other terms too.

The 2013 DSM-5 recognizes three types of bipolar disorder. Bipolar I disorder is characterized by depressive episodes and manic or mixed episodes that last one week or longer and have symptoms severe enough to require hospitalization. Bipolar II disorder is characterized by depressive episodes and hypomanic episodes, which do not cause impairment or psychosis, a break from reality. Bipolar II does not involve manic episodes. Cyclothymic disorder or cyclothymia is a milder kind of bipolar disorder and involves hypomanic and milder depressive episodes.

Edward Shorter's May 14, 2013, Oxford University Press blog, "DSM-5 Will be the last," discusses the problems with the classifications in the DSM-5. The blog points out there was no science-based reason for changing the name from manic depression to bipolar disorder.

Twenty percent of net proceeds from the sale of *Intact* will be donated to NAMI.

PART ONE

Trauma

"Many abused children cling to the hope that growing up will bring escape and freedom.

But the personality formed in the environment of coercive control is not well adapted to adult life. The survivor is left with fundamental problems in basic trust, autonomy, and initiative. She approaches the task of early adulthood—establishing independence and intimacy—burdened by major impairments in self-care, in cognition and in memory, in identity, and in the capacity to form stable relationships.

She is still a prisoner of her childhood; attempting to create a new life, she reencounters the trauma."

–Judith Lewis Herman, *Trauma and Recovery: The Aftermath of Violence - From Domestic Abuse to Political Terror*

CHAPTER 1

You'll Be in the Next Trash Bag

Spring 1978, Westchester County, New York

The gray sky lent an air of mystery to the Easter sunrise service about to begin. Tall, abundant trees surrounded me and nearly tricked me into thinking I had landed in a forest. The nearby reservoir resembled a lake. Trees, water, and the endless sky provided me with an invigorating dose of nature.

"We cannot live without hope. Nothing reminds us more than the promise and power of hope than the resurrection," said the pastor. His deep voice and the choir's hymns resonated in the fresh air.

"Just as the rebirth in nature is underway, hope can be reborn as well. Reach out for faith, and you will find it. It will renew you, grow within you, and restore your hope and strengthen your spirit," he continued.

His words replayed in my thoughts during my 30-minute walk home.

When I entered our apartment, I realized my father was still asleep. I made myself white rice and coaxed some clumpy cream of mushroom soup out of its can and onto the rice still in the pot and stirred them both until they blended together. With a bowlful of my favorite meal in hand, I headed to my bedroom to study. It was my junior year in high school, and I was determined to keep up my grades.

A few hours later, my father pushed open my bedroom door forcefully enough to create a breeze. By reflex, I put down the textbooks I had been studying in bed and stood up to greet him.

I could tell by his wrinkled forehead and tense stance that he was angry. "Your room is a f___ing pigsty. And you left your dishes in the sink," he seethed.

My father hated the sight of me studying while sitting in bed and repeatedly said, "If that's such an effective way to study, schools and libraries would do away with desks and chairs and have beds instead."

"Why can't you ever knock? I have no privacy," I answered. By the way his face became even more contorted, I realized I had said exactly the wrong thing.

"What the f___ do you need privacy for? You sneaky bitch." He lunged at me and hit me so hard I fell down.

Then he began to kick me. "I'll fix your ass. I'll show you how to clean up this mess," he sneered.

He left the room and returned with a hammer. "Go get some trash bags," he ordered.

When I returned to my room, I stood frozen as he used the hammer to smash everything in sight. My Fleetwood Mac albums became jagged shards of black vinyl never again capable of producing the sounds that comforted me and inspired me to choreograph interpretive dance moves.

He alternated between demolishing things and supervising my cleanup. He growled, "That's right. Pack up all this useless shit, so we can throw it out."

The only possessions spared were furniture and schoolbooks. There I stood watching—frozen like a squirrel stuck midway up a tree while a dog barks at it. There, but not there. Beyond emotion. Floating.

I began fantasizing about being at school and in ballet class. I told myself that what he was destroying were only things, and he couldn't touch my ability to make up dances, design clothes, or draw.

After he smashed my record albums, my camera, my collection of Royal Danish figurines, my miniature slot machine, and everything else in sight, his eyes rested on my high school yearbooks. Glossy pages filled with photos and crammed full of my classmates' year-end reflective notes and signatures became ragged scraps of black and white as he shredded my memories.

Still not satisfied, he went into my closet and ripped up my most cherished possessions, my antique clothing. Most of the 40s and 50s garments had been given to me by family and friends, and I had altered them to fit me.

I lost a piece of my identity with each seam that popped as he ruined my clothing. He unsuccessfully tried to rip apart a pair of lined wool trousers. He left the semi-ripped trousers on the carpet and stormed out of my bedroom.

Seconds later he returned with what looked like a diploma set in a white satin case. He ripped apart the case and the opaque, taffeta-like paper. His eyes became glassy with tears, and his voice caught in his throat as he uttered, "That was your mother's and my marriage certificate. It used to mean something to me, but now that I see what an awful slut you've turned out to be, I don't want it anymore."

When he was spun out, it would have been pointless to defend myself by pointing out to him I was a virgin and had not yet had a single date in high school.

He waved the remnants of the marriage certificate in front of my face before throwing them down. "She has it easy lying there in the ground. I curse her every day that she left you behind for me to raise. You're tainted. It must be your Swedish blood."

During his outbursts, he reminded me of my inferiority due to my Swedish ancestry.

His fury had exhausted him. He surveyed the mess with disdain. His screams became muffled as he yelled, "Clean this mess up. And don't try to hold on to any of this crap. Make sure you throw out all of these bags or you'll be in the next one."

For the first time, I feared for my life as he swung the hammer around, but I tried to deflect the vicious things my father had said to me by placing them in the trash along with my shattered possessions.

Mostly, I dealt with his violent outbursts by setting ambitious academic goals and blocking out what was happening.

CHAPTER 2

Meeting With High School Psychologist

One weekend, not long after Easter Sunday, I visited my father's Aunt Leah and her husband in a town on the other side of Westchester County. Their son had already coasted into an Ivy League college and onto its elite cross-country team.

After one night in their home, it was as if I woke up and became present in my body. Suddenly, I became aware of what had been going on at home. I felt the impact of five years' worth of beatings. I remember feeling jumpy and agitated and not wanting to go home.

I never wanted to face my father again.

I don't remember anything else except I ended up back at my father's home feeling defeated. I reverted to my old habit of blocking out his tirades and physical attacks by traveling elsewhere in my mind and picturing myself away at college.

As a child, when adults don't listen, you stop telling them what's bothering you. When I look back, I somewhat understand why my relatives became stuck in superficial. Growing up, I was well adjusted, an exceptional student, and had friends and activities. Why would one of my relatives want to rock the boat by dealing with my father and his explosive temper?

But inside, I was dying. My spirit was floating away. I had no way to make sense of the violence and degradation.

Even without abuse or neglect, many parents live through their children, because they value status above all else. They mold their children into a reflection of themselves instead of letting them become who they are.

English was my first-period class. My English teacher's theatrical voice bore the hint of a Southern accent. Even though he was, at most, 30 years old, some of the other Honors English students found him intimidating.

I found him intriguing. He made *The Great Gatsby* and everything else we read come alive.

One day on my way out of class, he said, "May I speak with you?" His question startled me. I wasn't behind in my work. I hadn't been disruptive or disrespectful.

By reflex, I answered, "Sure."

He got straight to the point. "Why have you been coming late to class?"

His question caught me off guard, and I answered, "I don't know. I am having a hard time waking up."

"You're so quiet. You're not yourself. You seem depressed."

"Depressed? I don't feel sad."

"Depression doesn't necessarily mean that you feel sad."

I don't remember the rest of the conversation, but I do remember feeling flustered and promising myself I would get to school on time.

My English teachers had been singling me out since junior high school and praising my writing, which always embarrassed me as I compared my writing to the authors we read in class and felt it fell far short.

I'm not sure how I ended up in the school psychologist's office. Did I miss a few days of school after spring break? Did my English teacher refer me? I remember little of our conversations during the few times we met, but I do remember a fragment of one conversation.

The psychologist interrupted me and said, "I just heard you say, 'I can't live like this anymore.'"

He added, "Did you hear what you said?"

He repeated what I had just said back to me once more and said, "Find a relative who will let you move in with them."

My mother's sister, her only sibling, lived in upstate New York. Less than a nanosecond after my asking her over the phone whether I could move in with her during my senior year, she turned me down. My aunt had been only 15 months younger than my mother and did not have any children of her own. Her outright, immediate, "No," stung.

Mor Mor and Aunt Leah each said I could come live with them after I turned 18. Eighteen was almost two years away and seemed like an eternity.

I felt abandoned.

My father's mother came from California to visit because she could hear how upset I was over the phone.

Several days into her visit, the three of us were eating dinner when my father lost his temper. When I stood up to get him something from the kitchen, he kicked me in my derriere, because I hadn't responded quickly enough to his request.

"I'm leaving. I can't stand to watch the way your father treats you," my grandmother said the next morning as I munched on Raisin Bran before leaving for school.

"Call me anytime," she added. Her panicked expression revealed her inner turmoil.

I don't remember any follow-up meeting after the school psychologist's recommendation. I can't ascertain whether mandated reporting was in effect in 1978, which requires teachers, counselors, nurses, and school administrators to immediately report suspected child abuse. Social services never got involved, which means my case was never reported.

I probably dropped off the school psychologist's radar, because I was a top student, had worked part-time as a high school lab assistant, was on the track team, participated in clubs, and had friends.

I had one year to go and was likely to get a scholarship to college. One year.

I had no idea there was a time bomb ticking away inside me.

CHAPTER 3

Scholarship Quandary

Spring 1979

I spent the summer between junior and senior year with my grandmother and my father's younger brother Uncle Mike in Southern California. Uncle Mike had seen how distraught his mother had been upon her return from visiting my father and me in the spring.

He tried to convince me to move in with him, "Come on, your high school has nothing on Wilson High School. I know you're worried about getting into East Coast colleges, but you'll have a better chance applying from a West Coast high school."

I was touched by his offer, but I had switched schools so often, I was hesitant to switch again, especially senior year, to a school in Southern California.

Spring of senior year brought college acceptance letters. I got into SUNY Binghamton and the three Seven Sister schools to which I had applied, but the slight slip in my junior year grades probably cost me admittance to Yale and Stanford. I didn't care. I was ecstatic to have been admitted to Smith College, my mother's alma mater, and almost immediately made up my mind to attend there.

My father was less than thrilled with my decision. He rattled off a number of reasons why Coracle College was a better choice and concluded by saying, "Coracle will look better on your resume."

Over the next few days, he alternated between pleading with me and expressing disgust that I didn't understand what should have been obvious to me. I finally gave in, because I was afraid of getting beaten up and couldn't handle the relentless pleading. After all, I would still be leaving home.

Our middle-aged guidance counselor had leathery, thickened skin. When I sat down to speak with him, I noticed the pale red and blue wispy veins on his cheeks. I only met with him once a year, but, even as a teen, I knew he looked like an alcoholic. When I met with him senior year, he said to me, "I can't picture you at Coracle. Don't you have some other options?"

I heard this same sentiment from several others, including an acquaintance my father and I ran into while walking through the grounds of our apartment complex. I had been admiring the trees in full bloom when the fellow mom approached us. She exchanged pleasantries with my father, and then she said to me, "Have you made up your mind to attend Coracle College? Somehow, I can't picture you there."

My father dismissed all of these comments as well-intentioned, but ignorant.

Senior year I don't remember meeting with the school psychologist. I didn't want to initiate a meeting—I felt ashamed. And I was counting down until I left for college.

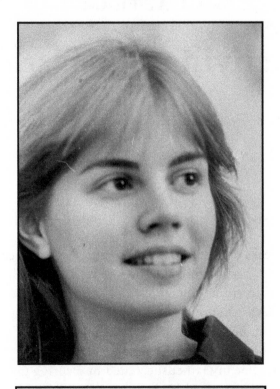

I was 16 during the fall of my senior year of high school.

CHAPTER 4

Reliving the Terror

Fall 1979

Within weeks of my arrival, Coracle threatened to revoke my scholarship, because of some rule about similar schools not being able to entice students with larger financial aid packages. My father was outraged because the scholarship was not financial aid, but an academic scholarship bestowed upon me by the school's Alumni Association.

By the time my father succeeded in securing my scholarship, my anxiety at the thought of losing it and having to return home to live with him ruined my idyllic college experience.

Striving to get a scholarship that would provide me with an escape from the violence and the indignity had kept me going for years.

Learning the classification of every living thing provided the sole curriculum for my biology class. Studying for exams involved memorizing detail after detail. The eight levels of classification quickly became eight levels of torture.

Right after Halloween, I received a C minus on my biology midterm and was devastated. I decided to quit the gymnastics club to give myself more time to study. Little did I know that was the absolute worst decision I could have made because my brain cannot concentrate without a fair amount of coordinated movement.

That tweak to my daily routine propelled me into an episode of immobility. I found it difficult to concentrate or talk or do much of anything. Daylight Saving Time didn't help my cause either, but I had zero awareness of circadian rhythms.

Looking back, every time I quit routinely exercising, depression followed. I did not realize there was a connection between exercise and mood. I didn't realize I needed exercise to help me concentrate and keep anxiety and depression at bay.

I woke up in the middle of the night startled to find myself in the top bunk in my dorm room and not in my high school bedroom. The dream had awakened me and seemed real, immediate. I had dreamed about a past confrontation with my father. He had been upset because I had put highlights in my hair in preparation for my vacation to Southern California and, at dawn, had made me carry my large suitcase two miles to the shuttle bus stop while kicking me from behind every few steps.

Once awake, my horrific memories were replaced with anxiety about flunking out and having to return home to live with him. I hated my biology and calculus classes and had no idea how I would pass them. In high school, I had been blessed with gifted teachers who made themselves available every day after school and who made their curriculum come alive.

I must have gotten back to sleep, but I woke up exhausted that morning. Throughout the morning, fragments of the past night's dream invaded my thoughts as did memories of the occasional "frozen" days I had had in high school. Along with entering high school at 13, after yet another move, had come monthly periods. Often, for about a week around the time of my period, I would become lethargic, have difficulty concentrating, and become unable to block out my father's erratic behavior. During track season and when I took ballet classes regularly, these symptoms had disappeared, so I hadn't given those unusual days much thought until that awful feeling of incapacitation returned.

After lunch, I headed toward the library and found an isolated cubicle amidst the third-floor stacks. I opened my biology text and tried to study, but the words jumbled. While trying to memorize the classification of every living thing, I was losing my ability to describe any living thing.

I reached for my flashcards, but the details would not stick. If I couldn't visualize it or figure it out, I couldn't remember it.

Some of the other students kept saying, "This is easy, all you have to do is memorize everything." But my brain couldn't memorize scads of facts and details, only concepts and formulas I could apply.

I switched to calculus, but I had to read the directions to each problem ten times to grasp its meaning. The humming sounds of the pumped-in white noise at my college's library became an adversary. The white noise invaded my slowed thoughts.

Time dragged. My thoughts echoed over and over in an endless loop, and I felt conscious of my being, of my existence in space. An hour passed, and I had only halfway completed one calculus problem.

After dinner, I again attempted to study for my biology test. I lay on my top bunk in my dorm room studying the chenille pattern of my bedspread and looking at my watch every few minutes. Each time I told myself, *In fifteen minutes, I'll get up and go to the library.*

By the end of the semester, I had visited with the school psychiatrist, Dr. Ivy, and she had arranged for me to drop second-semester calculus and biology. She believed, and I came to believe that the episode of depression I was experiencing was solely responsible for my inability to pass those classes.

College science and math are different than high school science and math. Although I had to study a lot in high school, I loved algebra, geometry, and probability and statistics and did quite well in those classes. Second-semester calculus is different. It's four-dimensional. It's beyond analysis and logic. I could not grasp it. Period. Perhaps if I spent 10 hours a day on that one subject, I could have passed the class, but there are not enough hours in the day to spend 10 hours every day on one subject. It was not my strength.

My short-term memory retrieval is not good, nor is my ability to memorize lots of detailed information. I grasp concepts, big ideas, quickly and can effectively write about them. I had placed myself in the wrong majors, pre-med Biology and then Chemistry.

My grades were my identity. Losing my ability to attain them, despite tremendous effort, crushed me.

My father had been averse to my attending a large state school because it didn't have as much prestige. However, at a large state school, there would have been more majors as well as more mental health and academic counseling resources.

There is more to this story than the disassociation that enabled me to survive the pain of child abuse and bury it in my subconscious. There is wiring. You can influence your brain circuitry by building new neural pathways through your actions and habits. However, if you're not musically inclined, no amount of practice will turn you into a concert pianist.

Many years later, I learned about how important it is for someone with bipolar disorder to accommodate for shaky circadian rhythms.

I now realize I experienced significant changes to my routine between high school and college. I had many opportunities for physical activity in high school. I walked for miles every day, cleaned the apartment and cooked, ran track (except for senior year), took dance lessons, and practiced and made up dances for hours every week.

When I left for college at 17, I also had no clue dance and drawing had been my "creative outlets." I first took ballet classes from the age of four until five. I fell in love with connecting to music through movement and practiced on my own nearly every day. Because I didn't have access to dance lessons for years at a time, I took to choreographing dances on my own. My father wasn't home much, which meant the sparsely furnished apartment became my dance studio almost every evening.

I danced my turmoil away. I didn't realize dance had served as my therapy too.

CHAPTER 5

Circadian Rhythms and Bipolar Depression

A lot of research points to the link between bipolar disorder and having a faulty circadian rhythm, the 24-hour internal clock controlled by the hypothalamus that affects hormonal cycles, body temperature, and the sleep/wake cycle.

"Circadian rhythm in bipolar disorder: A review of the literature" was published in the September 2018 issue of *Psychiatry and Clinical Neurosciences,* and its abstract summarizes key points about the link between them:

- "Sleep disturbances and circadian rhythm dysfunction have been widely demonstrated in patients with bipolar disorder (BD)."

- "Irregularity of the sleep-wake rhythm, eveningness chronotype, abnormality of melatonin secretion, the vulnerability of clock genes, and the irregularity of social time cues have also been well-documented in BD."

- "Circadian rhythm dysfunction is prominent in BD compared with that in major depressive disorders, implying that circadian rhythm dysfunction is a trait marker of BD."

CHAPTER 6

Dream Date

New Year's Eve 1979

Adam had starred in my daydreams during high school even though he had a girlfriend when we met. He attended a neighboring high school. We met at a Model United Nations when I was in 10th grade and he was in 11th grade.

My senior year in high school was his first year in college at Columbia University in Manhattan. He was 16 when he started college, and his youth caught up with him. He had gotten off to a rough start, including experimenting with speed. His wavy blonde hair had become shoulder length and unruly. I didn't care. I adored him.

We kept in touch and got together a few times during my senior year, but after graduating from high school, I spent the entire summer in Southern California with my uncle and grandmother.

During the Christmas break of my freshman year, we reconnected. New Year's Eve Adam and I walked for an hour and a half through snow-covered roads accented by evergreens, which resembled giant Christmas trees. His worn jeans always fit in all the right places, and he walked lightly on his feet.

His arm felt like it belonged around my shoulder. It was a crisp evening. Everything looked clearer. Everything sounded better, particularly Adam's moderately husky voice. Listening to his voice filled me with warmth.

He had turned 18 a few days earlier, and I was to turn 18 in a few weeks.

We arrived at his friend's party just in time for the midnight toast ushering in 1980, the new decade, and to watch the televised broadcast of Blondie performing "Dreaming." Deborah Harry mesmerized the entire room as she commanded the stage, managing to look sultry dressed in a multi-zippered khaki jumpsuit, a couture version of a Department of Sanitation uniform.

I didn't let go of Adam's hand all night or stop looking at him. His yellow-blonde hair wisped around his neck and the sides of his long face, which still bore traces of acne. When he smiled, his face appeared to be all dimples and his blue eyes smiled too.

An hour or so later, his friends drove us to his home. We entered to find his mother sitting in their large, brightly lit kitchen paying bills. "Did you have fun?" she asked.

For three years I had settled for being Adam's friend. That night was our first true evening date. To kiss him and hold him in my arms the entire evening filled me with such joy that I could barely speak. I nodded my head idiotically while Adam described the party.

"Sasha will sleep in Jeannie's room," Adam said as he guided us out of the room. I caught his mom amusedly rolling her eyes.

By dawn, we had been making out and cuddling for what seemed an eternity. Adam looked so comfortable without his clothes that his tall, slender body didn't seem nude. I remember searching for the right words. I wanted to tone down my enthusiasm and sound somewhat offhand. I finally blurted out something to the effect, "I feel ready. We won't get many chances."

He sighed and said, "I know we've known each other a long time. I am very attracted to you, and I really like you, but I am not sure I am in love with you."

I felt crushed. I wanted to respond, *But I am in love with you,* but instead, I said, "I know how I feel about you. I'm crazy about you and have been for three years. I thought you felt the same way."

"You're a virgin and your first time should be about love."

I rubbed my body against his, took his hand in mine, and said, "I certainly can't force you."

He laughed and hugged me, "Well, it wouldn't be a bad thing for you to learn to be more patient. You're always in such a rush."

After New Year's Eve, we saw each other a few times over the break, and I got a chance to visit him in his dorm room in the city. We returned to kissing and holding hands. I had made my willingness to go further beyond obvious, and I didn't want to be pushy and make our brief time together uncomfortable.

CHAPTER 7

No One Was Listening

January 1980

During Christmas break, my father had traveled to Europe
to marry a European doctor whom he had met in October.
She had been working in a major New York City hospital as
a visiting specialist. I took advantage of his absence to move
in with Aunt Leah, but when he returned, he threw a tantrum
and threatened to cut off my money for textbooks.

Sometimes he didn't follow through, and I didn't panic
until the semester began and he did follow through. I was on
academic probation and lost in my math and science classes
even when I had textbooks. Within 10 days, my panic sur-
passed anxiety and verged on hysteria.

In 1980, there was no Internet and there were no e-books.

A few of us were hanging out in the dorm living room made
cozy by the discarded furniture that had ended up there.

"The answer to everything here is to throw a tea party," I said. Everyone within earshot howled with laughter. I wasn't trying to be funny. I was trying to make sense of a culture I did not understand. I had lived for weeks and sometimes months in several European countries and Southern California and attended school in three different states and three entirely different neighborhoods within New York City. Throughout high school, I had passed for a college student and attended numerous adult events with my father in Manhattan.

I had been hanging out at college campuses since I was born. Never in my wildest dreams did I consider that the culture of a college campus would mystify me.

I suppose I mystified the college's administration even more.

Most of my classmates came from elite private schools in which the culture was restrained and understated during the day at least. I had grown up among many cultures, but the real me was direct, sincere, and silly. I had discovered my true nature during my brief time in Paris and all the time I had spent in New York City since junior high school. It didn't hurt that a fast-talking charmer helped raise me.

I was much more expressive than my Coracle classmates. I had grown up around New Yorkers who elevated exaggeration to an art form with their expressions and body language and relatives from my father's side of the family who gestured frequently and greeted each other by kissing each other's cheeks three times.

My anxiety and effusiveness as I attempted to communicate with Dr. Ivy must have alarmed her the two or three times I met with her, because, in the fall, I had been lethargic and inarticulate.

I was used to not being listened to. When Dr. Ivy rifled through her notes and changed the subject when I broached the subject of my father's abuse, I stopped trying to get through to her.

The trauma was raw—six years of my handsome, witty, and brilliant father frequently transforming into a violent bully who would degrade me, bang my head into the wall, destroy my possessions, and worse. At the time, the violence I had experienced at the hand of his otherwise attentive mother from the ages of three to seven seemed insignificant.

At the age of five, I had starved myself for months during my time with my father's mother. During high school, I had become a binge/starve eater, and during my first semester of college, the binging and starving became worse. But, in the 1980s, how you ate was generally not thought to have anything to do with anything except your jeans size and whether or not you should wear a bikini.

Three weeks into the semester, I became overwrought when trying to explain to Dr. Ivy that I would not be able to pass my classes without textbooks.

"Take good notes in class, and see if you can find some of your textbooks in the library." (Of course, none of the textbooks I needed could be found in the library.)

Again, I felt as if she were dismissing me. I did not yet know I needed to put on an act with her, endure her, until I could find someone capable of listening to me.

I respected her. I trusted her. I felt awful, and I wanted to feel like myself again. I had no idea what had been at stake—that with the stroke of a pen, she could diagnose me with a condition that would rule out entire careers and affect my ability to get certain types of insurance for the rest of my life.

As a young adult, starving myself with crash diets could precipitate episodes of panic and agitation. Because my bulimia was relatively mild, I did not consider that there might be a connection between how I felt and what I ate. Dr. Ivy never inquired about my daily habits, such as the way I ate.

Nor did she suggest I take an interest inventory or see an academic counselor when I hit the wall with biology and second-semester calculus.

Around most of my classmates, I slipped into my persona and must have appeared carefree most of the time.

On a Thursday night toward the end of January, I was obsessing about my schoolwork and Max, the guy I had begun dating the week before. It was too early in the semester for students to be pulling all-nighters. By 11 p.m. I found myself alone in the dorm's living room watching TV at a low volume and soothing myself with Tabs (diet cola) from the dorm's vending machine, not realizing that the caffeine in them upped my anxiety and made it difficult for me to sleep. I finally fell asleep around 1 a.m.

On my way to breakfast the next morning, the freshman dean showed up, which seemed strange, as I had only met with her in her office. I was on one of my ultra-low-cal diets and hadn't eaten more than a handful of calories in 24 hours. I had achieved "hangry."

The dean, whom I doubted was capable of ever achieving hangry, said, "I need to take you to the infirmary. You can have breakfast later." She delivered me to the infirmary and said good-bye.

"Did you sleep in your room last night?" Dr. Clark, the doctor who ran the infirmary, asked. Her pearly, cat's-eye framed glasses had lenses so thick they magnified her eyes. They resembled fish eyes.

Her question uneased me because I thought it was her roundabout way of finding out if I had a sex life. I didn't have the blood sugar level to politely answer, *Yes*. Instead, I responded, "I don't think that's any of your business."

Her mouth puckered as if she had sipped rotten milk. "Did you sleep at all last night?"

"I didn't sleep long. I had a lot on my mind."

The more questions she asked, the more indignant I became. She had made me miss breakfast, and I was hungry. My morning class was about to begin, and I resented her for keeping me from it.

When she told me she didn't think I was fit to be in college, I felt as if my integrity had been attacked. I shouted, "Leave me alone."

I felt hated, and I could not verbalize my thoughts, *I want to study—I just don't have the books. Lots of students pull all-nighters. Why was I being singled out for having slept six hours the night before? Why was everyone pretending it was no big deal not to have textbooks?*

She left the examining room and returned with a pill and a paper cup of water. "Take this. You need to rest," she said firmly.

By reflex, I swallowed the capsule and then asked, "What is it?"

"Thorazine. It will help you relax," she said and then escorted me to a corner of the infirmary. "Please make yourself comfortable here, but you cannot leave the infirmary. Someone will bring you breakfast shortly," she said before retreating.

That morning I had unwittingly subjected myself to the everyday habits that cause me to panic and become anxious and irritable. Caffeine late at night. Fasting and super lo-cal diets. Interrupted sleep. No matter how many years stable I have been, my blood sugar and my mood remain closely linked. That took me years to discover on my own.

Amy, my best friend, immediately came to visit me. Her ankle-length, red flannel nightgown adorned with tiny teddy bears peeked out from under her long navy wool coat. Amy and I caught up while sitting on the edge of the twin bed in the nearly barren infirmary room. She, along with most other students, found Dr. Clark laughable and was alarmed that my fate rested in her hands.

Right after Amy left, Dr. Clark introduced me to the first of my round-the-clock private nurses the school had hired to watch over me, "Catherine this is your nurse, and she'll be helping us out today." Although my legal name was Catherine, Sasha had been my childhood nickname and the name I had my friends call me. My mother had given it to me when I was one year old. We had lived in Eastern Europe for about nine months while my father pursued graduate studies there, and I had been told she heard the name and liked it.

The only reason for the nurse was to ensure that I did not set foot outside the infirmary. It was beyond strange to me to know someone was being paid to guard me.

The day became more surreal because the Thorazine caused my body to betray me. My mouth became so dry that I gulped down a pitcher of water every hour. At least filling my cup gave my private nurse something to do.

The sunlight that penetrated the glass-walled waiting room, my cage, made my eyes ache and tear. Changing position caused my joints to stiffen and throb.

Amy spread the word about my imprisonment. A steady trickle of visitors throughout the day made me feel a little better.

Early Saturday morning Amy came to visit again. She was trying hard to cheer me up and said, "Lawrence, Chris, and Brandon came to visit you last night too. Right after dinner. Lawrence was upset. He tried to wake you up by sitting you up and shaking you. He said you were like a rag doll. That it was eerie. Like you might never wake up. What did they give you?"

"Thorazine, whatever that is. What a nightmare. I worked so hard for so many years to get into a good college, and after a few months, my entire future is gone. It's not fair. Like I'm still in my father's shadow," I moaned.

"Sweetie, you must have faith in yourself." Amy took my hand in hers as if trying to will her determination for a happy ending into me.

"I have faith in you, and I love you very much," Amy said. She was interrupted by Dr. Clark who entered the sick room and said, too cheerfully, "Your family's here and Dr. Ivy's here, so why don't we all sit down and talk together in the waiting room."

Everyone spoke at once. My 83year-old Mor Mor looked startled, my Aunt Leah looked disgusted, my stepmother looked shocked, and my father looked irate. The moment I saw my father, I burst into tears.

Dr. Clark wore a lopsided smile. Dr. Ivy, clad in jeans, looked calm but grim.

When I heard plans being made for me to return with my father, I stood up and screamed, "I'm not leaving with him. If I have to live with him, it would kill me."

Before I could explain that I meant it would kill my spirit, Dr. Ivy urged me to calm down and ushered me into an empty office to speak with me privately, "I know you'd rather go home with your aunt, but your father is your legal guardian. Your only other option is to stay in a nearby hospital for a short time until we can work out your living arrangements."

Three weeks of trying to study without textbooks, the shock of being under house arrest, and the effects of Thorazine had worn me out. I could not register my primary emotion, betrayal.

In one day, why had my doctor arranged my imprisonment in the infirmary, talked to my father, my abuser, behind my back, prescribed me horrific tranquilizers, and suggested I leave college without bothering to consult me?

"I'll go to the hospital," I said resignedly.

We walked back to the waiting room where my father was ranting at Aunt Leah about his father's will. Students were trickling in and out of the infirmary and walking right past the waiting room.

My entire drama had been played out in front of any number of my classmates.

Pain and Rage

Spilling out
Spilling in

Come undone
Again, and again

Pretend it's not happening

Survive
Numb

Came to believe
That I don't count

No one listened, no one cared

Be quiet. Carry on.
You're such a smart girl.

CHAPTER 8

Locked Up

January – February 1980

Dr. Ivy accompanied my father and me to the metropolitan hospital that accepted my father's health insurance. The intake interview was less involved than opening up a checking account. A form materialized for me to sign. The form stated that I was voluntarily committing myself and taking legal responsibility for myself. A couple of weeks before, I had turned 18. It should have occurred to me, that at 18, I had legal rights and could have gone home with my aunt, but I was so used to being a minor, it didn't.

My father was asked if he had anything to add. Tears pooled in his eyes as he said, "Perhaps I was too hard on her. I never meant for this to happen."

A nurse took me down a carpeted hallway and showed me to my room. I put my few things in the closet. When an aide brought me a dinner tray, I resisted the impulse to tip her.

I felt as if I had checked into a hotel.

Walking past the locked doors of my upstairs ward made me realize I was not just in any hospital, but a mental hospital—the very place my father had threatened to send me in the worst of his rages. Overnight, my dreams had disintegrated, and I feared being stigmatized as a mental patient for the rest of my life.

The hospital was clean and well-kept, although drab. It was remarkable in its ordinariness.

The great majority of the patients appeared ordinary too, although most of them smoked incessantly and complained nonstop. At least a quarter of the patients had ended up in my ward because there was no place else for them to get treated for their drug or alcohol addiction. The nurses were pleasant and addressed me in a normal tone of voice, unlike one of the doctors who spoke to me slowly, as if I had the IQ of a salamander.

Spending 24 hours a day with the other patients in my ward meant everyone quickly learned the highlights of everyone else's history. The other patients were familiar with my college, and a number of them called me snooty and stuck up. One fast-talking, tall, Black man in his late thirties sought me out in the lounge and said, "I've been studying you for days. You don't belong in a hospital."

Aware that he had my full attention, he paused and said, "You know what your only problem is? You read too much."

Sunday, I called Aunt Leah collect and told her about the hospital. She said, "Well, I'm glad you still have your head on your shoulders. No one bothered to tell me what happened or where you ended up."

"I miss you so much, and I can't believe I'm not still at college," I said avoiding the frowns of the other patients lined up to use the payphone.

"You sound so good. Sasha, you have your whole future ahead of you. Try to hold your head up high, and be strong.

You'll make it through this. I promise you," Aunt Leah said in her firm, clear voice.

Monday morning arrived along with Dr. Ivy's familiar face. "I want to help you. I don't want you to have to live with mood swings anymore," she began. All I could do was listen.

She spoke as if she had rehearsed a speech, "When we first met, you were extremely depressed. You've told me that you have suffered for years from depressive episodes. Your recent agitation indicates to me that you suffer from manic-depressive illness.

"Irritability and not being able to sleep are some of the symptoms of the manic phase of this illness. You need not feel hopeless. This illness is highly treatable. With the proper medication, you can lead a normal, productive life."

"Medication, I don't have to keep taking Thorazine, do I? It makes me feel awful. When they weighed me this morning, I've somehow gained seven pounds since Friday." I could feel the denim of my jeans cutting into my thighs.

"You're probably just retaining water. You'll only have to take Thorazine a few more days until the lithium starts working. You will have to continue taking lithium when you leave here and get regular blood tests to make sure you maintain the proper level in your bloodstream." The low pitch and monotone cadence of Dr. Ivy's voice rarely varied.

"I won't get depressed anymore?" I asked.

"Not like before," Dr. Ivy promised.

Dr. Ivy's diagnosis didn't bother me at first. Manic-depressive sounded poetic. My few brushes with depression scared me, and I looked forward to never having to deal with depression again.

I only saw Dr. Ivy a handful of times for a few minutes at a time. All I could think about was getting out of the hospital.

She never brought up my fear of my father or the abuse I had mentioned once. She didn't seem interested. I was so used to the pretend game, that I didn't keep trying to explain the flashbacks, the nightmares, and the constant dread that I would never break away from my father's control.

Once I got a diagnosis, it was as if my genetics were responsible for everything awry in my life, and only the proper amount of medication could remedy everything.

My initial journey into the mental health system broke my spirit and traumatized me further. I had survived the beatings, threats, and contempt by compartmentalizing them, by listening to music, by studying incessantly, and by binging and starving.

Upon diagnosis, I lost my identity.

Dr. Ivy was not unkind or incompetent, but this was the early 1980s, and she was narrow-minded. She did not believe that what had happened to me, no matter how violent or traumatic, had anything to do with the diagnosis of manic-depressive illness she bestowed upon me. She believed that medication alone was the only answer and the highest recommended dose at that.

Half the patients seemed as if they belonged in rehab and others needed more attention than the hospital could provide. There were at least three other teenagers out of the thirty-odd patients in my ward. One of them didn't seem to belong there. Mark had bushy dark brown hair and a high forehead. He spoke eloquently. When silent, Mark always appeared to be intently concentrating, as if he were on the verge of solving some obscure calculus equation. He also played the piano with such feeling and prowess.

Mark told me he had been in schools for the emotionally disturbed since junior high school and that he hated being so sensitive. "I can see through people. I can see things most people can't, and it's been that way since childhood. I feel what others are feeling, and mostly it hurts to feel so much."

"But Mark, that's a gift. That's what makes you an artist. I do know what you're talking about.

"When I was 11 years old, we visited my cousins for a couple of weeks. I astounded my uncle with my insights into his neighbors. He told me I noticed things most adults never noticed, and I realized I was different."

A look of recognition flashed through his sad eyes, "You do understand. Almost nobody does."

"But you can't focus on that all the time. You need some release, like your music. That's why I love to dance. That's the only way I survived living with my father." An image of him slamming me into a wall caused me to wince for a moment.

"But I'm afraid I'm not as strong as you are," he sighed as he resumed playing the piano.

I tried to befriend Sarah, a 19-year-old from a state college in New Jersey, but she was shy. The ugly scar around her neck served as a constant reminder that she had almost succeeded in killing herself. Looking at it triggered a mental image of her passed out in a pool of dark red blood as more blood trickled from the gash in her throat.

Every weekday the entire ward, patients and staff, met for a brief morning meeting. One tiny, middle-aged, alcoholic man always bugged me to hold my teddy bear, Horatio. I knew I was too old to carry around a teddy bear, but he was plush and small, immensely huggable. Aunt Leah had given him to me for Christmas to replace the many childhood possessions my father had smashed and destroyed during his rages.

Someone had noticed me crying while I had been talking on the payphone, and it was discussed round-robin at the meeting. I felt as if I were a freak on display. I had been talking to Amy about Coracle activities that had once included me.

I had been crying because I felt as if I had been edited out of my own life.

I had been crying because I felt as if I had been edited out of my own life.

37

Max was amazed at how I spent my days going from one group therapy to the next. During one of our phone conversations, I said, "Guess what? Today in occupational therapy I made you a monkey out of socks, sort of a mascot for your room."

"Thanks."

"And then in movement therapy today," before I could finish my sentence, Max cut me off.

He said, "Movement therapy! What does your movement therapist teach you? How to take a shit?"

While I had been confined to the infirmary, my roommate, upon request from the school administration, had hastily thrown together some personal belongings of mine. A half-empty suitcase full of underwear and not much else had been delivered to me. I dictated to Max a list of additional items to collect from my roommate. Fleetwood Mac's album *Tusk* was the first item on my list.

Max seemed like so much color against the grays and whites of the hospital hallway. I was embarrassed to have him see me in the hospital setting. At a loss for words, I led him outside to the patients' small garden area and kissed him furiously. For that moment, I felt like myself.

Our time alone was short-lived as a security guard ushered us inside.

Stevie Nicks' voice didn't sound quite as haunting from the portable record player in the rec room as it did on a stereo system, but the textured, evocative music soothed me because it reminded me of life outside the hospital.

Most of the other patients hated *Tusk*. One evening, a perpetually worried-looking older woman ran out of the room with her hands over her ears proclaiming, "If I have to listen to that one more time, I'll really go nuts."

Food numbed me. Even the odorless, colorless hospital meals became appealing—instant mashed potatoes, rubbery chicken, overcooked vegetables that fell apart upon contact with the fork, and sweet, pasty pudding that gagged me. Food that normally killed my appetite now slid down my throat.

We also received two snacks daily, just as in nursery school, which were usually juice and stale, generic-brand cookies not capable of crumbling. Keeping painfully full and torturing my taste buds distracted me from feeling much else. More hospital privileges meant I could supplement my five feedings a day with vending machine and hospital cafeteria food.

One day I ran into Joan, a fellow patient, in the cafeteria. A sixtyish woman with the posture of an army sergeant, a stiffly hairsprayed updo, and the demeanor of a prison guard, Joan had recently stopped parading the halls with her walkie-talkie. No one had ever figured out who she thought was at the other end of the walkie-talkie.

Joan frowned at me, "You've put on a noticeable amount of weight in a short time. You've got to control yourself. It's a crime for a young girl like you to be fat."

I listened to her as I demolished mini-donuts which blanketed me with white sticky powder and tasted like sugar water. I wiped some powder from my chin and mumbled, "You're right," praying she would shut up before she completely ruined my appetite.

Around dawn of the day before my discharge, one patient killed himself by hanging himself with the belt from his bathrobe. He had been pale and fading, incapable of casting a shadow.

His pain had been so overwhelming, it had surrounded him like a force field. His medication had not worked.

The Other

No longer elite
Off the path
At best, ordinary

CHAPTER 9

Overmedicated

1980

During my hospital stay and upon release, I did not receive any therapy to cope with a childhood marred by physical, mental, and emotional abuse from the ages of three to seven and 11 to 17. Nor was I given any insight into how to take care of myself other than to take an amount of medication that lowered my blood pressure to 90 over 60 and made me so light-headed I could not keep from nodding off all day long.

After the hospital, I ended up back in my father's apartment for a few months, and one of the first things I did was visit with my minister. The church, built in 1869, was only a 15-minute walk from our apartment. It was a striking piece of architecture that featured perfectly chiseled pale gray stone arranged in symmetrical patterns and stained-glass windows framed by mosaics of small silver and dark gray stones.

The minister ushered me into his office. It was the first time I had had a private meeting with the slender, white-haired minister. After I recounted a brief summary of the hospitalization, the normally enthusiastic, energetic minister bristled and said, "Well, there are county mental health services."

And that is all he said.

His body language was stiff. He looked uncomfortable. He looked as if he wanted the conversation to end.

I felt as if I had been shoved down to the ground. I was speechless. This was the gifted orator? This was the man who conducted prison ministry at times? I had been an integral part of his church for four years, and he couldn't even offer me, a floundering 18-year-old, a few words of comfort or welcome me back to church services?

The science of the brain itself is far too complex to ever be absolutely exact. Having pored through studies in many medical journals and books, such as the best-seller *Moodswing* first published in 1975 and authored by Dr. Ronald Fieve, a psychiatrist who was a pioneer in the effective treatment of bipolar disorder, I was able to follow the research trail and determine what had been established by what year.

In the 1980s, not as much was known about bipolar disorder as is now, but some major insights had been established, such as the critical need for regular sleep, how effective exercise can be for managing mild to moderate depression, and that nutrition can play a role.

Although the right dose of lithium works magic for me, too much lithium creates a nightmare for me.

The amount of lithium I was prescribed at the time made my blood pressure drop to an alarmingly low level, which made me tremendously dizzy and prone to passing out. I also had difficulty speaking at times as the words would not emerge, but Dr. Ivy would not adjust the dose. Dr. Ivy and most other medical doctors are not trained in addiction medicine, and my eating disorder was not recognized as an addiction or considered significant.

Too much lithium can flatten you. The dose of lithium I was first prescribed made me feel weak and light-headed. Not awake. Not asleep.

And then there was the lithium static constantly reverberating in my head like an endless almost-headache. My appetite went into overdrive. I quickly gained twenty pounds.

I hated dragging so much weight around.

Eventually, the recommended therapeutic dosage of lithium was decreased. The study, "Decreasing lithium dosage reduces morbidity and side-effects during prophylaxis," published in the November 1983 issue of *Journal of Affective Disorders* cites fewer side effects and other benefits from a lower dosage.

"Lithium Treatment Over the Lifespan in Bipolar Disorders" published May 7, 2020, in *Frontiers in Psychiatry* says, "Preventing new episodes in BD is essential with regard to quality of life, participation in society and preventing long-term disability. Lithium remains the gold standard in achieving this goal. It is effective in both type I and type II BD."

How many individuals diagnosed with bipolar disorder respond to lithium? That is hard to assess from the research. My experience has been that medication is rarely enough.

Can you drive a car with no fuel in the tank? Can you avoid anxiety and depression while living on caffeine and chocolate and being dehydrated?

Unless other lifestyle variables are taken into account that might allow a particular medication to work, it is hard to assess the efficacy of a medication.

CHAPTER 10

Buried Pain

1980

During the spring and summer that followed my disastrous freshman fall semester, I met with Dr. Gray, a psychiatrist recommended by a friend of mine's father who was a psychiatrist himself. I only met with Dr. Gray a few times. He was a kind man who listened to me, except by then I had shut down.

He suggested that I go through childhood photographs to trigger memories and to reconnect with former feelings. I sifted through photos and felt nothing.

That last year of high school with my father I had survived by shutting something off, my pilot light, and I couldn't reignite it.

I didn't register a sense of loss looking at photos of my former stepmother and brother whose absence I had mourned for years.

When I was seven, my brother was born. After his birth, I moved from Manhattan to a storybook college town in

Wisconsin to live with my father, my brother, and my brother's mother.

During the college semester, my father would often sequester himself in his study or disappear. In his absence, my stepmother, my brother, and I bonded.

My brother almost felt like my child, and right then and there, at seven years old, I knew I wanted to have children one day.

Unfortunately, when my brother was two and a half years old, my father abruptly split up with my brother's mother, and she moved across the country and then back to Europe.

None of my father's abuse registered either, even when I looked at photos in which my body language and expression displayed distress.

Nor did looking at photos of myself dancing rekindle feelings about expressing myself through dance or some related creative outlet, such as drawing or designing clothes.

Even when I looked at the photos from the film taken from my mother's camera after she died, I did not feel any longing for my mother or wonderment at how she had captured her three-year-old daughter, me, joyously jumping and playing in a huge pile of rust-colored leaves.

No reaction to a photo of my five-year-old self, nearly skeletal, from starving myself for several months.

No horror registered at the photo of the first-grader who had gone from practicing leaps to sullenly staring.

No remembrance of all the years of beatings.

The trauma of the hospitalization and the all-consuming fear that I had lost my ticket out of Hell trumped the abuse, which I had been successfully blocking out for years anyhow.

At 18, all I could feel was the strong desire to get back into college and redeem myself with good grades. My entire identity and self-worth rested in my grades.

I weaned myself off of lithium again sometime in the spring, because I didn't see why I should have to take a medication every day which caused me unpleasant side effects when my depressions were few and far between. And I hated the 20-plus pounds I had gained. I didn't recognize myself in the mirror. Even worse, I didn't recognize my body—I felt awkward and slow as I walked.

I couldn't reconcile my grave diagnosis with who I was.

Passing twelve weeks of chemistry lectures, labs, and tutorials at NYU's summer school earned me another chance at Coracle College.

Since saying good-bye to lithium, I was down to 145 pounds. Only 10 extra pounds remained. Thinner, I walked differently. I loved pressing my feet into the ground and taking longer, more forceful strides.

Back then, I did not realize that the ratio of muscle mass to body fat was far more important than weight.

The semester started great. However, memorizing formula after formula for my Organic Chemistry mid-term and trying to solve calculus equations zapped me. After a while, the equations would flip. I was used to occasionally transposing numbers and not being able to tell left from right. However, Organic Chemistry became an undecipherable code. I did not know I had slight visual processing challenges, let alone how to accommodate them.

I resumed taking lithium, but that did not make Organic Chemistry or Calculus any easier.

While at a dorm party on a Saturday night, I noticed a young woman with long, wavy red hair standing next to a tree and talking to herself. She looked disheveled. I realized I had seen her off by herself before, silently crying, so subtly, that it had only registered to me that she had been crying after I had already walked by her.

I walked over to an acquaintance and asked, "Who is that? Is she all right?"

"That's Cecily. You don't need to worry about her. Her father is a powerhouse attorney. She does this a lot."

I vaguely remember going up to her and making inane small talk to distract her from crying, but my memory is so hazy, I can't be sure that I did.

The next day, it occurred to me how nonchalant the partygoers had been about Cecily. Whereas, when I returned to campus, my friends had told me all the rumors there had been about me—that I had slapped Dr. Clark and that I had tried to commit suicide. At the time, those rumors hurt deeply, but as I neared the end of the semester, failing half my classes, the mystique of the school had worn off. I was beginning to imagine myself elsewhere.

I finally realized why several acquaintances had tried to talk me out of attending Coracle. In essence, it was a finishing school. You went there to get into graduate school, meet a suitable rich husband, or make the connections to work in a prestigious low-paying job, in publishing or in a museum, that necessitated tapping into a trust fund. It was a small liberal arts college with few majors, and it certainly wasn't the place for someone trying to discover a career outside of academia, law, art history, or medicine.

Most of my classmates were classy and friendly. Many of them had graduated from prestigious private schools. My disconnect was with the academics. The classes were either too easy and not at all challenging or indecipherable.

One of my male friends from Coracle's brother school said to me, "College is all about going through motions. You expect too much."

I flunked both Organic Chemistry and Calculus, which translated into flunking out of Coracle College and losing my scholarship.

CHAPTER 11

Q&A Interview With Dr. Laryssa Creswell

Long-Term Effects of Childhood Trauma

Laryssa M. Creswell, Ed.D., MT-BC, LPC, LCPC Operations Manager/Therapist-Empowered Connections, LLC, Adjunct Professor–The Chicago School of Professional Psychology, Washington DC

Q: How does trauma lead to disconnection and disempowerment from others and from self?

A: Judith Herman in her seminal book, *Trauma and Recovery: The Aftermath of Violence from Domestic Abuse to Political Terror*, explains that when a person experiences a traumatic incident, it calls into question all of what was understood or known to be about people around them and their environment.

That experience severs all of what was known about who they are and who they are within the world around them. Therefore, disconnecting them from relationships whether family, friends or significant others, their community, and life. They become disempowered by the lack of sense of control and understanding of what has happened to them and the world around them.

Q: How does trauma lead to co-occurring disorders?

A: I view trauma, mental illness, and substance use in a triad. One can potentially lead to the other or stand on its own and not connect with the other. There can be many variables that could be contributing factors but will be different for each individual person or in this case specifically individual woman.

Mary Ballou and Laura Brown in their book, *Rethinking Mental Health & Disorder: Feminist Perspective,* challenge the clinician to account for various societal "isms," (for example, classism, sexism, and racism) when trying to understand what has led a person to substance use.

When we know that the traumatic experience has a direct link to substance use and/or mental illness and have an understanding of the individual person's lived experience, a more specific course of treatment can be established.

Q: Why should trauma be assessed at intake?

A: The assessment should occur at intake to have a full understanding of the person's life experience at the point of entry to ensure proper and comprehensive treatment is provided. Best practices would be to use a "universal precautions" approach which would require treatment providers to consider every person sitting in front of them as possibly having experienced a traumatic event.

Additionally, without assessing for trauma at intake, symptoms observed could be understood improperly and lead to misdiagnosis which in turn could lead to treatment being provided that is not effective.

Additionally, without assessing for trauma at intake, symptoms observed could be understood improperly and lead to misdiagnosis which in turn could lead to treatment being provided that is not effective.

Q: How can using trauma as a framework for treatment lead to more effective treatment of bipolar and other mental illness?

A: According to the Substance Abuse and Mental Health Services Administration, there was a time when trauma was thought to be an unusual experience. Now, it is understood that exposure to a traumatic experience is considered to be a more common issue, with 60.7% of men and 51.2% of women having experienced at minimum one trauma within their lifetime.

Trauma-informed care (TIC) ensures that a survivor will encounter providers who believe that trauma has a pervasive effect on an individual's physical and mental health. By practicing TIC, this ensures that necessary services are provided to move an individual towards their highest potential. Traumatic experiences can play a part in the manifestation of other diagnoses.

Trauma-informed care should be at the forefront of a clinician's mind to do no further harm. When trauma is taken into consideration from the beginning of an individual's matriculation through services, the clinician is more likely to develop treatment that is comprehensive and meets the specific needs of the individual.

PART TWO

Chaos

"What is addiction, really? It is a sign, a signal, a symptom of distress. It is a language that tells us about a plight that must be understood."

–Alice Miller, *Breaking Down the Wall of Silence: The Liberating Experience of Facing Painful Truth*

CHAPTER 12

Nineteen

January 1981

In March 1981, I moved to Long Beach, California to live with my father and stepmother. My father, bored with his previous career, had become a commodities broker. One of his clients was a local psychiatrist. This client became my new psychiatrist.

At nineteen, I did not understand the difference between a therapist and a psychiatrist. Having flunked out of college for the second time, I felt like a slug. Not truly alive. A mistake.

My new doctor prescribed lithium at a lower dosage and it did help give me the energy to enroll in summer school, work a part-time summer job, and enroll in Cal State Long Beach through their Extended Education Program.

October 1981

Halloween fell on a Saturday in 1981, and I fell hard for Andreas, a Norwegian exchange student I met at a Halloween party. I had not been in a romantic relationship for close to a year.

Within a week, my anxiety escalated as I fixated on whether he would become the love of my life or simply a bittersweet memory. I began having trouble sleeping and sitting still.

My new doctor prescribed the benzodiazepine Ativan, a minor tranquilizer, and another benzodiazepine that can be used as a sleeping pill, Dalmane.

Ativan wipes out your anxiety in totality. For a few hours.

Within weeks, I craved further escape and began smoking weed, a drug I had not touched since the age of 13.

After breezing through a philosophy class in summer school, I had felt comfortable enrolling in 15 units, a full load, of general education classes. By staying on top of my assignments that fall semester, I was getting good grades until the last third of the semester.

Falling in love proved to be torture. I could not concentrate nor could I sit still. Nor could I rest within my own skin. My heartbeat and pulse quickened.

School was all I knew. Once again, the anxiety over not being able to make it through the semester made it feel as if someone had put a gun to my head.

Pills, weed… nothing could relieve the pressure enough. Although I had had sex on only one occasion prior, with Max, I began an affair with an acquaintance, Andreas' friend, because it provided a temporary escape from the unrelenting pulsing and non-stop thoughts. Before the end of the semester, I also slept with another acquaintance after becoming so drunk I felt as if I were floating above my body.

I ended up receiving a medical withdrawal with the option of taking my finals after winter break.

In retrospect, I can track my episodes by the calendar. As spring turned into summer my mania would emerge. Right around Daylight Saving Time at the end of October, severe depression and anxiety overtook me. This, my first full-blown manic episode, was the only one that happened in the winter.

I did not know then that it would be 18 years before I would gain any insight into addiction, functional addiction, and trading addictions.

December 1981

Needing a break from another hellish semester, I made plans to travel to New York City over Christmas break so that I could visit my relatives in New York City and the few high school friends with whom I was still in touch.

However, on my first Saturday night there, I set out alone for Studio 54. My newfound need to travel with as many accessories as possible meant I couldn't use any of my purses because they held little more than my wallet and keys. I shoved make-up, perfume, reading material, my Walkman, and Mary Janes into a small blue TWA flight bag. Struggling to decide which of two shirts to wear, I donned the striped burnt orange polo one and threw the oversized royal blue one into the flight bag.

Before heading to the subway, I checked myself out in the mirror and admired the way my new color-blocked light green, cream, and beige ski jacket matched my iridescent Sassoon jeans that went from metallic light green to beige depending on how the light hit them.

It was pleasantly crisp, a reprise from the wind-chill factor that made the wind so cold it penetrated my temples and made my head throb. On my way to the club, I stopped at a deli to have some tea and fell into conversation with the young

Omar Sharif look-alike working there. By my last sip of tea, I learned that he was Turkish, a part-time model, and that he wanted to get together at 2:30 a.m.

There was only a short line at Studio 54, which was located in a marginal neighborhood formerly known as Hell's Kitchen, 54th Street and 10th Avenue. The club was about as far west as you could go without ending up in the Hudson River. The entrance was unimpressive aside from the velvet ropes and the bouncer who looked as if he had stepped out of a J. Crew catalog.

The club was late opening and my face burned from the wind and the cold. I approached a guy in a dark gray sharkskin suit who had been walking in and out of the club and said, "I'm supposed to meet my boyfriend here later, and he'll be upset if I get any more frozen." I touched my overly rosy cheek and pouted, "I don't know if my face will recover in time."

Suit Guy suppressed a snort, but he did escort me into the club while the rest waited. I entered the club by walking through a black hallway disguised as a tunnel. My rationalization about the fictitious boyfriend story was that it was only partially a lie because I would have no chance of meeting any potential boyfriends with a wind-burned face. The lie had easily rolled off my tongue. Normally, I was incapable of lying. Even telling white lies made my pulse race. My father had often accused me of being "compulsively honest."

The winding tunnel opened up into a cavernous, glittering nightclub with infinite nooks and crannies. Everywhere I turned, a different bar was being set up. Even empty, the purported pleasure palace took my breath away. I took advantage of the deserted club and slowly danced solo on the gleaming hardwood dance floor.

A couple of hours later, I teamed up with a ravenhaired beauty, Tracy, who was also 19. She was classily attired in an ivory silk blouse and black wool pants. Our mutual interests—men, modeling, and partying—guaranteed our immediate rapport.

That night was the first time I heard a serious DJ in action. He sped up, slowed down, and repeated sections of songs to make them more danceable. The strobe and other lights were manipulated in rhythm with the remixes.

The pulsing lights enhanced the superior sound system, as did the special effects, such as fake snow and silver streamers emanating from the two-story ceiling.

Many areas and atmospheres were contained within the vast layout of the club, and I had fun discovering each one. There was an upstairs bleacher section with its own bar, a never-ending dance floor, and various clusters of sectional vinyl chairs, sofas, and cocktail tables randomly distributed throughout the club.

Like clockwork, at 2:30 a.m., I left the fantasy world of Studio 54 and my new best friend to meet with Riaz. He kept telling me how beautiful I was and that he couldn't believe he had met me. It was hard to believe compliments repeated ad nauseam, and I irritably snapped, "Shut up." My tone startled him into compliance.

Riaz had promised me breakfast in the Bronx, where he lived, and he delivered. We devoured eggs, potatoes, and pancakes galore. Then we returned to his apartment and he showed me his modeling portfolio. I asked him how often he worked, and he replied, "Not too much. It's harder to be a male model, and it doesn't pay as well. But you should get into it. You'd only need to lose about ten pounds. Then your body would be the perfect type."

I groaned, "I know. I weigh 140 pounds, and I can't get any lower."

"I'll help you."

Shortly thereafter, we were thrashing around in his small bed. Heat blasted from the radiators and made us sweat even more profusely. In between gasps, I thought to myself, *I don't want to be here, and I can't believe I am having sex.* It was as if I had stepped on an express bus when all I had intended to do was cross the street.

It was as if I had stepped on an express bus when all I had intended to do was cross the street.

When I woke up after a short nap, it was still morning. Riaz walked me to the subway and waited with me until I caught my train. He offered to help me move my things from California to New York, and I promised to call him as soon as I could.

Minutes later I realized I'd never call him. Riaz was a stranger. By the time the subway pulled into the Bay Ridge station, that realization didn't bother me. Riaz no longer existed.

At 19, I had slept with my first stranger, but by lunchtime the next day, it didn't register. My behavior had been a complete departure from my very essence. Mania, fueled by the drugs that had escalated it, destroyed my character. It robbed me of my judgment. It robbed me of me.

But mania wasn't my only adversary. Compulsive-addictive behavior complicated matters, but, at 19, I had zero insight into how it played into the equation. Within his book *Bradshaw on the Family,* acclaimed educator and author, the late John Bradshaw defined compulsive-addictive behavior as "any pathological relationship with any mood-altering experience that has life-damaging consequences."

While manic, while lacking judgment, while lacking a filter to my overwhelming impulses, while hormones raging, very little of me remained.

Those two months, approximately Thanksgiving time until the end of January, represent my first true manic episode.

Hysteria, nightmares, my inability to process the years of abuse, and not having a proper place to live had landed me in the hospital days after my 18th birthday.

At 19, prescription pills had triggered my craving for marijuana, which research suggests can hasten manic episodes.

Mania

Anxiety...

paralyzing
mobilizing

Short-circuiting reason

Panic, desperation, indecision
Oh, so wrong decision

Impulsivity
Judgment impaired...
Gone.

CHAPTER 13

Intersection—Rock Musician

1983

There's a major intersection in Long Beach right before the intersection in which 2nd Street turns into Westminster Boulevard. It has one of those traffic lights that lasts for minutes. As I waited there, I noticed a gorgeous young man waiting to cross the street and spontaneously asked him, "Would you like a ride?"

It was late afternoon. He turned to me with a quizzical look on his face, which appeared alert and honest. Excellent posture.

Somehow, I was not afraid as he smiled and said, "Sure."

Rock-n-roll music blared from my speakers, which kept the conversation to a minimum. It turned out Jim had recently gotten out of the military, did not yet have an automobile, and was riding the bus to get around. He was 23 to my 21.

We ended up at my studio apartment not far from downtown Long Beach. Meeting Jim felt like amazing luck, and I didn't want to break the spell. I rushed to the stereo and played a song that matched my mood, David Bowie's "Sound and Vision."

"I can't believe you know that song," he said with a shy smile.

Jim was so relaxed, he made me feel at ease. We kept listening to songs. My studio apartment was small, and eventually, we ended up sitting next to each other on my bed.

I lay down because the music sounded better that way. He stroked my hair as he gazed at me. If I had two words to describe Jim, they would be kind and gentle.

Unable to control my racing heart and the tingles overtaking my body, I sat up and kissed him on his mouth.

He looked at me amusedly and we began kissing for real.

Jim was a gentleman. We kissed for a long while. It was I who was intent on having sex.

In three short years, I had gone from not wanting sex to interfere with my future goals to using it as a way to pass time.

All I remember about that first time is it felt really good. Cozy, comfortable, as well as erotic.

When it was time again for conversation, Jim revealed, "I put together a band. I took a job at a motel so I would have time to get something going with the music."

I admired Jim's focus. I was already up to my fourth major, economics. My inability to memorize copious amounts of detailed information took me out of biology and chemistry. Although I could churn out sketches of highly original concepts, illustrating umpteen versions of them was simply too tedious, which had ended my would-be art major.

Jim and I were hanging out on a weekend night with some of his music business friends in one of their home studios. I had been smoking weed and was pleasantly high. Some song played that compelled me to sing. I belted out the lyrics and shocked everyone in the room.

"I didn't know you could sing," said one of his friends wearing a just-faded-enough, just-zippered-enough black leather jacket.

I laughed and shrugged in response. Little did they know, I could only sing like that when I was wasted.

That had not always been the case. I had loved to sing along to rock-n-roll songs ever since first grade and would beg for 45 singles as gifts. In eighth grade, my friends would goad me into getting high so I could pretend to be the lead singer and sing along to rock-n-roll standards, such as "Honky Tonk Women."

Right before ninth grade, my father and I moved to Westchester County, New York. In ninth grade, I auditioned for the high school chorus.

The music teacher appeared to be in his early sixties. He called us in one by one. I didn't feel nervous, but the notes that came out of my mouth sounded hesitant and faint.

The music teacher ran his fingers up and down the keyboard prompting me to match the notes he played.

After I was done, he looked perplexed and said, "Nobody has a range of three notes. I have never seen anything like this."

When had I lost my voice? By then, at 13, I had been living alone with my father for two years. Losing my voice marked the beginning of losing my identity and my connection to my spirit.

Jim loved watching me dance and would say, "It comes so easily to you. You would look so good on stage. The way you move."

I didn't know then that I had stage fright so severe it paralyzed me. How can you explain to someone else what you can't even acknowledge to yourself?

Jim was creative and determined to make a living with music. Those qualities drew me to him, but my lack of focus frustrated him as did my inability to take music seriously. He saw my potential as a lyricist and back-up singer and dancer. My spaciness mystified him, and after a few months he dumped me, but we remained friends for several years.

I wasn't manic when I met Jim. I wasn't depressed. I wasn't on any medication either. But, at 21, I was without a tether. In high school, I had been completely focused on earning a scholarship. There had been no stopping me. I worked exceptionally hard at school, at dance, and at drawing.

Drive and discipline are my strengths, but focus has always been my challenge. However, when I do zero in on something, my focus becomes intense.

Setting daily, short-term, and long-term goals has been the main way I deal with my struggle with focus.

Setting goals helps me block out distractions. At 21, I didn't realize this.

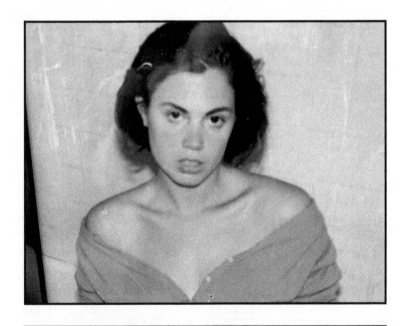

Under the influence. Summer 1983, probably.

CHAPTER 14

Stranded on the Freeway

Summer 1984

The deserted freeway's brightly lit lanes appeared to be immaculate. I was on my way to visit Jim, who still worked a graveyard shift at a motel in Garden Grove when he wasn't performing rock-n-roll. A couple of exits before my destination, I ran out of gas and steered my car onto the shoulder.

Within minutes, a gray-haired man dressed for the golf course pulled up in a van and offered to drive me to a gas station. He looked like a young grandfather. I hoisted myself and my satchel of belongings into the front seat of his van.

As he merged back onto the freeway he asked, "Where are you headed tonight?"

"I got into a fight with my roommate and was on my way to visit a close friend who works nights."

He took his eyes off the road as he turned toward me and said, "Hey, can you show me your tits?"

"No."

He kept trying to grab me as he drove, and I noticed he seemed jittery as if he had been doing coke.

"Let me out of your car," I screamed.

He stopped near an off-ramp. While I squeezed through the van's partially open door, he stepped on the gas.

As I flew into the midnight sky, I instinctively tucked my head and body into a forward roll before slamming into the pavement.

Not sure if I was still on earth, I lay winded and in a heap on the shoulder of the off-ramp.

When I attempted to stand up, my right hip throbbed as if shards of glass were piercing it. The front seam of the hem on my denim skirt was frayed, and my legs were scratched and bleeding. My face stung and I could feel scrapes and cuts too. My oversized satchel containing clothing, my purse, phone book, and ID had driven off with the van. I guessed that I was still in Orange County.

Underneath a black sky beginning to turn gray, I limped off the freeway and kept limping until I saw a 24hour coffee shop. Bright fluorescent light greeted me. A waitress wearing a vaguely 50s uniform materialized across the freshly waxed beige linoleum floor. I asked her to call the police for me. Her mouth hung open as she gaped at me and said, "Sure honey. Are you going to be OK until they get here?"

I nodded my head before collapsing into a booth. Seconds later the waitress returned and said, "They're on their way. Anything I can bring you?"

"Just some ice water please," I answered and then proceeded to hang my head and silently cry.

Within minutes, two police officers arrived and slipped into the booth with me. Still choked up, I tried to tell them what had happened, "My car ran out of gas on the freeway. Some harmless looking gray-haired guy in a van offered to drive me to get some gas."

I gulped down the glass of ice water and felt a jolt as the cold invaded my body and made my head throb slightly. "He kept trying to fondle me, so I told him to let me out of the car.

"He stopped by an off-ramp, but as I opened the door, he must have put his foot on the gas, because I went flying. He must have done it on purpose because he sped off."

"What kind of car was he driving?" the faceless police officer with the notebook asked.

"I don't know. It was a white or off-white van."

"Did you see what make it was or get a partial plate?"

"I'm sorry, but cars all look the same to me, and I was upset to begin with because of being stranded on the freeway." I took another swig of water and began chewing an ice cube.

"Can you give us a better description of him?"

"Well, he was in his late forties. He had a full head of gray hair. He was dressed in nice casual clothes and had kind of a round face."

"What kind of clothes?"

I tried to picture him. "Umm, off-white chinos, a polo shirt, and a windbreaker."

"What color shirt?"

"Yellow, I think." The officer had stopped taking notes.

"I'm going to be honest with you. I think you invented this entire story, because you tried to harm yourself by jumping from somewhere, and you are trying to cover for yourself. You don't remember enough details," he said sounding bored.

"What are you talking about? That's crazy."

"Calm down. OK, answer me this. Why are you wearing two different color shoes?"

"Because the heel of the turquoise pair is broken, and I was in a hurry tonight. I grabbed the red one because they're the same shoe in different colors," I said as I realized that my fashion statement had probably cost me my credibility.

"Well, we don't have enough information to look for the van driver, but we will drive you to the hospital so they can x-ray you."

The officers escorted me to the emergency room of UCI Medical Center. The hospital seemed completely white and new. A nurse immediately attended to me. She briskly moved me from a waiting area to the x-ray room and then to an examining room. The policemen lingered, traipsing along with us and continuing to question me.

The nurse helped me climb onto an examining table. The police officers stood on either side of the table. One of them said, "You must remember more details. Did he say where he was headed?"

A middle-aged doctor strode into the room and took in the scene. He walked right up to one of the policemen and firmly said, "You need to leave the examining room." Something in his tone made them comply. They both nodded at him and quietly walked out without a word to me.

The x-ray arrived. The doctor studied it and said, "Your hip is dislocated. This is going to hurt," and then proceeded to pop my hip back into place. My scream sounded louder than I thought a human scream could sound.

"You're lucky you didn't break any bones and your injuries were minor. Your hip is going to hurt for a while. It's going to be painful to walk, but I suggest you do," he instructed and then took off.

The nurse cleaned and dressed my cuts and scrapes. She tended to the cuts on my face last. When she was done, another nurse informed me that no one had answered the phone at any of my three friends' homes.

"Aren't there any family members we can call to pick you up?"

"No." She took me over to meet with a social worker who questioned me while attempting to fill out a form with my information.

"Where do you live?"

"Uh, I'm kind of not sure."

"I don't understand," she said sounding annoyed.

"I was subletting a room, but I can't live there anymore."

"Are you currently employed?"

"I go to college. I quit my last part-time job a few days ago."

"I see." She paused, "What about family?"

"Nobody I trust."

"Surely there is one relative we can call who can come to pick you up." She looked over my bruised and cut body and sighed, "You're in no condition to travel."

"No one. I'm sure," I said with finality. My family members were still furious that I had moved out, and I was terrified that assistance from any of them would lead to an ugly confrontation with my father.

She shoved the almost blank form aside. "Well, we can't force you, but I think you need psychiatric help. We can't hold you today, but please get some help soon."

Her remark made me furious. *Who was she to judge me?* To keep myself from screaming at her, I struggled out of the chair and hobbled out of the office.

Once outside I noticed a waiting police car, and one of the officers gave me detailed directions as to how to get to Long Beach. After several blocks, I rested on a bus bench. Unsolicited, an elderly man handed me ten dollars for food and bus fare before boarding his bus. From the corner of my eye, I glimpsed a Mexican restaurant and spent the entire ten dollars on tacos and enchiladas. The food gave me enough energy to resume walking.

While I walked, I kept trying to figure out how I was going to rescue my car and navigate my way back to Long Beach. The intense afternoon sun gave me a headache. My throbbing hip began to feel as if it was being sliced open, and I sought refuge in a park by sitting on the lawn under a large tree.

Neither asleep nor awake, I was dreamwalking.

I became aware that someone was talking to me. "You sure look like you've had a rough day." The words belonged to a slight thirtyish man dressed in navy work pants and a pale blue work shirt.

"I ran out of gas on the freeway early this morning. Some man offered to take me to a gas station, but instead, he attacked me. He sped off when I was exiting his car, and I hurt my hip and got scraped up."

"Well, you might be in luck. My name is Steve and I have a small towing company. I'd be happy to take you to your car with the tow truck. My office is right near here. We can walk there," he said.

We left the busier streets and wound around fenced-in dirt lots to get to the tow truck company that turned out to be a tiny, shabby office with an attached room and bathroom. The room was furnished with a desk, a couple of chairs, and a single bed. All the walls were in need of a good scrubbing. The brown-black industrial carpet was worn thin.

Steve pointed me toward the bathroom, "Why don't you wash up while I make some business calls." Before I could answer, he disappeared into his office.

The bathroom's toilet was in its own closet-sized room. The sink and vanity area were located outside it. I made a beeline for the toilet and then came outside to the sink and tried to clean my arms, legs, and face without disturbing the salve on the cuts. It was the first chance I had to study my face in a mirror. The cuts made my face look as if it had been patched together. One deep jagged cut obscured my chin. I was sure I'd have scars.

Steve returned and turned on a small television. "Geeze, even your clothes are torn. I have some old stuff here you might feel more comfortable in," he said.

I gazed down at my torn denim skirt. The largest rip was fraying. While I considered his offer, he produced white jeans and a dark blue Hawaiian shirt that looked as if they'd fit. I changed in the toilet room. When I emerged, Steve was sitting on the bed smoking. He offered me a cigarette, which I accepted.

One cigarette led to another and Steve was absorbed watching inane TV reruns.

"Shouldn't we get going?"

"I'm waiting to hear about a job, and then we can take off. Why don't you come and sit next to me on the bed," he casually suggested.

"I had better get going." My hip throbbed as if a wrench had found its way inside my hip socket and was twisting my hip bones round and round. The pain radiated all the way down my leg.

Like a cockroach exposed to bright light, Steve ran to the glass door. He produced keys from his pocket and locked and bolted the door. "It's double-plated bullet-proof glass. Don't even think about trying to break it," he growled.

He turned his back, and I lunged toward the door anyhow, in desperation thinking maybe I could unlock it somehow. Before I could make any progress, Steve was behind me pressing me into the door and putting what felt like the cool, thick blade of a hunting knife next to my ear.

"If you don't listen to me, I'll cut you."

I realized how much I wanted to live and silently prayed to God as I pleaded with Steve.

"I'll do whatever you want, just please don't kill me." Steve eased the knife away from my ear and steered me toward his bed.

What Steve wanted was sex, oral sex for starters. He also wanted me to act as if I were seducing him. Queasiness overtook me, and I gagged at the thought.

"Look my mouth is all cut up, and my jaw is throbbing. Couldn't we just have sex?"

Steve looked at me with disgust. "Listen you rotten whore, you're turning me off. You better take your clothes off, and you better make it sexy."

I kept from grimacing as I took off my clothes by picturing myself safely out of his clutches and nightclubbing with friends. When I was nude, he ordered me to lie on the bed while he removed his pants, underwear, and shoes. Wearing only his grease-stained work shirt, he pinned me down and thrust wildly like a pigeon flapping its wings.

He kept repeating, "Does it feel good? Come on baby, I want to see you orgasm." I faked an orgasm by gasping, moaning, and moving my head side to side, a terrible job, but enough for him to finish off.

He immediately climbed off me, dressed, and adopted a neutral tone of voice. "You really are a prostitute, aren't you? This is nothing for you?"

He'd say something else but kept coming back to trying to make me confess I was a prostitute. Finally, I said, "Yes."

"One more time and I promise you can go," Steve said. He repeated his crude brand of intercourse with me, got dressed, and handed me $60, which I refused to take. "Here, now I've given you what I owe you, but you can't leave until you take the money."

I realized my pride could cost me my life. I took the money and said, "Thank you." He was quiet as I dressed, but true to his word he walked me to the door, unlocked it, and released me into the night.

My injured hip kept me from running, but I walked away as quickly as I could while tears streamed down my face. The howls of guard dogs echoed my pain and shock.

Within a block, I threw the three $20 bills into the wind. As I watched them swirl and blow away, I was released from sicko Steve's spell.

After walking a couple more blocks, I turned onto a side-walk bordering a six-lane street and attracted the attention of another man in a car. This man looked to be my age. He had short dark hair and a clean-cut air. Somehow, his good looks reassured me. His face could easily have adorned an Air Force recruiting poster. He drove an old well-kept Lincoln or Cadillac.

The driver pulled up to the curb and asked, "Are you OK?" I couldn't answer. I couldn't stop crying.

The driver, concerned, persisted, "Where do you live?"

"Long Beach," I sputtered.

"Let me give you a ride home," the stranger said as he opened the car door. Without responding, I climbed into the car.

I didn't say a word for the half-hour ride until we approached Long Beach, and he asked me where he could drop me off. I indicated the shopping mall where my gym was located and thanked him for the ride. Once inside my favorite nightclub, I headed straight for the bathroom. That night I was immune to the alternative music, the retro wood paneling, the soft lighting, and the life-sized paintings of Bogart and Bacall. Crowded inside a bathroom stall, I changed back into my clothes and attempted to flush Steve's clothes down the toilet.

My head felt warm. To cool off, I ran the water from the sink until it felt icy and then splashed it on my hair.

I had attempted to give myself a shag haircut after getting high the day before. Jagged spikes were all that remained of my bangs. Wet, the spikes looked like porcupine spines. I washed my face over and over, trying to avoid all the cuts, as I contemplated my next move. I hadn't recognized anyone inside the bar but remembered that an acquaintance of mine, James, was probably waiting tables a couple of short blocks away.

I hobbled from the nightclub to Hof's Hut, a cozy coffee shop, and spotted James. Tall and lithe with a distinctly graceful walk and skin the color of cappuccino, he was easy to spot. He took one look at me and pulled me aside.

"I had a huge fight with my roommate and then was in a minor car accident. I can't face my family yet. I'm too upset. Could I sleep on your couch tonight?" I didn't want to discuss the rape. I wanted to forget about it as quickly as possible.

"Of course. I have to get back to work, but I'll be finished in an hour. I'll find a quiet booth for you where you can wait for me," James said as he set me up with iced tea and a newspaper.

Class act that he was, James did not ask me any questions, other than would I be OK when he dropped me off the next morning near my roommate's apartment.

CHAPTER 15

NA Meeting

1985

None of my friends or acquaintances attended Narcotics Anonymous, NA, or any other 12-step meetings. I am not sure what inspired me, at 23, to walk through the door of a hospital meeting room that was hosting an NA meeting other than the realization that my drug use could get much, much worse, because I loved getting high, and I had made my second trip to the psych ward the summer before. I was also becoming aware I had become dependent on prescription pills to manage my anxiety.

Ativan worked wonders in the short term, but it kept me from developing any recognition of the early symptoms of depression or hypomania, not-quite mania, such as irritability and distractibility. (Hypomania, by definition, does not cause impairment or psychosis, a break from reality.)

It's much easier to deal with a low-level symptom than it is to deal with one that has escalated.

In eighth grade, together with my friends in Queens, New York, I had experimented with weed, hash, and PCP on weekends.

The summer after eighth grade, I had quit cold turkey, because I had witnessed some of my older friends graduate from making out to sex and from weed to heavier drugs, including acid. I hadn't wanted to do the same. I hadn't touched another drug until being prescribed benzodiazepines at the age of 19.

What kept me coming back to the NA meetings were the relaxed atmosphere and the feeling I was surrounded by genuine people who cared about each other. I didn't relate to most of their day-to-day lives as most of the other attendees were middle-aged and had consistently abused drugs for years.

I did relate to the tales of heartbreak. Breakups left me feeling hollow and bereft. My sense of self was so fragile that when my relationships didn't work out, there was no me left to come back to.

Even though the term 12 steps were entwined with Alcoholics Anonymous and all its spin-offs, the steps themselves were hazy to me. When I heard them read out loud, they made sense to me, but I had no concept of what it meant to work steps.

Because my usage was intermittent, I was not sure I belonged and did not attend often. I did not connect the dots between smoking weed and mania or alcohol and mania. I did not view alcohol as a drug.

I had no insight into addiction and that it could morph from one substance to another or from a substance to a behavior. I did not connect my torrid relationship with food with influencing my emotions or with addiction. I simply saw it as a failure of will power or discipline.

CHAPTER 16

Washington Square Park Dealer

Summer 1988

During a summer vacation visit to Mor Mor, I found myself walking through Washington Square Park in Greenwich Village. The park setting reminded me of a lazy afternoon spent there with my middle-aged distant cousin Peter while I had still been in high school. He had been visiting from Denmark, and the park had been one stop during a whirlwind day touring Manhattan. We had watched a street performer, self-styled stand-up comedian Charlie Barnett, create a sizeable audience out of tourists and others strolling through the large park famous for its commanding marble arch styled after the Arc de Triomphe.

The park was almost as renowned for having drug dealers available 24/7. Sometimes, you can tell by how they whisper or signal to their clients. Sometimes, you can tell by the way they sit and watch. On alert. Sometimes, you just know. And, sometimes, they let you know. Like that day.

Speed is what I wanted. Cocaine is what I got.

I don't remember the walk back to my hotel room or how the drug dealer ended up back there with me. Most likely we had fallen into conversation, and I hadn't noticed that he was walking with me.

In the privacy of my hotel room, I finally snorted my purchase. Feeling absolutely relaxed while at the same time feeling completely awake overcame me almost instantly. "This is different. I think I like it."

Before I could mentally catalog exactly how it differed from speed, Park Dealer approached me. I thought he was getting ready to leave, but instead, he pulled me out of the cozy faded mauve velvet-like armchair and dragged me toward the nearby bed. He instantly overpowered me, and my struggling proved to be useless.

He raped me so quickly that I disassociated for those few minutes and didn't feel a thing.

As soon as he was done, he left.

Later that evening, I began to have trouble breathing. It felt as if my throat was closing. It didn't seem as if there was much room left in my throat until I would be unable to breathe at all, and I wondered if this was to be the end.

Shortly after we met, Park Dealer had written down his phone number in case I needed a fix. I debated calling 911, but I was not eager to reveal what I had been using. Instead, I called his number. A young woman answered.

I blurted out, "I'm having trouble breathing. I am scared."

"It's an allergic reaction from the coke. It will go away," she reassured me.

"Are you sure?"

"It's not uncommon. You're going to be all right in a few hours. You are not going to die," she said reassuringly.

She continued, "Call me back later if you need to." Her sincerity calmed me down, and the breathing scare temporarily made me forget about having been raped. I took my allergic reaction to the coke, or whatever it had been cut with, as a sign to stick to weed.

Going Out

Don't care.
Don't stare.

Go away from me.

Me is gone

I no longer know you
Don't want to know you now.
Don't want you to see me now.

When I'm straight,
I will return.

CHAPTER 17

Exit Runway Left

Summer 1988

Over the phone, Aunt Leah took care of turning my airline voucher into a return ticket to LAX. I took a bus to the airport and boarded the airplane bound for Los Angeles.

While waiting for takeoff, I looked out the window and wondered what it would be like to work at the airport. I reached for the airline magazine, but all I could find was a catalog of useless gadgets.

I looked around the airplane. The passengers and flight attendants seemed to be moving in slow motion. The plane looked like a movie set.

I felt a strong pull toward Manhattan, even though I no longer had a place to live there. An editorship at the school newspaper awaited me in Long Beach, and I only had a few classes to go until graduation. I loved reporting and writing articles. I had been pursuing a diploma on and off for nine years, yet it was as if a magnet had pulled all logic and sense of self out of my brain.

A sense of urgency overtook me because I had a primal need to be away from my father. Some force was propelling me to stay in New York, and I summoned a stewardess. I must have looked stricken because she didn't question me when I told her I felt ill and could not make it through the flight.

I walked off the plane.

Summer

Bummer
Should be funner

Long days
Exciting nights

Off the rails
Mind sails

CHAPTER 18

In Harm's Way

September 1988

"Shut that bitch up," said Pops from the front seat of a 1970s Chevy Impala (my best guess as to the make of the car).

Serge, my latest intstaboyfriend, grabbed my shoulder, twisted my torso toward him, and punched me in the mouth. Pain emanated from my teeth and through my jaw. A welt, a cross between a cold sore and a blister, took over my lower lip. No man had hit me since my father.

The night was fading into gray dawn when we arrived at the building they called a hospital. It was surrounded by a barren field of yellow-brown grass—a setting straight out of a Kafka novel or a slasher movie. The building was several stories high and vast. I looked around for a sign with the hospital's name but didn't find one. There were several empty lots of land adjacent to the "hospital." The neighborhood resembled some kind of industrial area because there were alleys and factories in the vicinity.

We weren't in Manhattan, but I had no idea where we were. Zamir, the driver who had claimed to be an FBI agent, wandered off with Pops whom he insisted was his father. I got out of the car and yelled at Serge, "How do you know Zamir?"

Serge glared at me.

I continued, "How could he be an FBI agent and drive like such an asshole?"

Nothing I said elicited a response from Serge. He leaned against the car, his body rigid. His eyes looked at the pavement, anywhere but at me. He smoked a cigarette. Another cigarette.

Finally, he stepped on the butt of his cigarette and stared at me. The face looking at me was the face of a stranger, alert and together. His features looked more exaggerated and in sharper focus. He looked more like a cop than an artist. Silently, he walked away toward the "hospital."

When he was almost to the building, I belted out a classic rock-n-roll tune, desperate to get his attention. I improvised some of the lyrics, "Pleeeaaassse, honey, please don't leave me now. I'm begging you down on my knees. Don't you dare tease." He disappeared around the side of the building.

My heart crashed along with the rest of me. Speeded up no longer, I felt faint, weightless, as if an unlikely breeze in the humid air could blow me away. My eyes felt as if someone had been sanding them. For several days, I had survived my miserable circumstances by consoling myself with the thought that I had met the man of my dreams, and now he was abandoning me. Whoever Serge was, he had treated me horridly. Still, I waited by the car, urgently hoping he'd return.

Ten minutes later Zamir showed up by himself. I asked him where Serge was, and he responded, "I promised you a ride back to Manhattan. Get in the car and I'll take you."

I got in the front seat and kept asking him questions about Serge to no avail. As we drove, anxious to break his silence, I switched approaches and asked his opinion of my favorite celebrity. Zamir answered, "Brilliant. But he takes too many chances, unnecessary chances."

Zamir drove into an alley and stopped the car. It was still early in the morning, and the entire area was deserted. I thought he was stopping to pee in some nearby bushes. Instead, he said, "There's something you have to do before I take you any further."

I wondered what I could possibly do for him. He exited the car, came around to my side, opened my door, and grabbed my hand. "Come on, we're going in the back seat," he said firmly.

He shoved me into the back seat, got in himself, and said, "I want to have sex with you."

I prayed I could fast-talk my way out of the situation, "No, I can't. You know Serge, and that bothers me. Besides we just met. I don't have any condoms. You're a young, good-looking guy. You can get lots of girls. You don't need me."

"You're making such a big deal out of nothing. Come on. You need a ride, and I need a release. Trust me. You don't want to be stranded here."

We squirmed around in the back seat as he tugged at my clothes and pinned me against the car door. With all his weight pressed against me, I could hardly breathe.

Fully clothed, he raped me. Every time I panted for breath, the windows fogged up more and more, and I thought he would somehow smother me to death.

When he finished, I was dazed and didn't want to be near him. "Let me out of the car." He happily complied and drove off.

I tried to get my bearings by walking, but I felt torn. It was as if my insides were dripping out along with his semen.

I found myself in an abandoned field with grass that reached up to my shoulders. I followed some trampled grass and ran into a crack addict futilely trying to inhale crack from an empty metal pipe that resembled plumbing hardware. He threw the pipe at me and muttered something unintelligible.

His balance, his muscle tone, and his IQ had been smoked away, and I easily got away from him. I thought to myself, *If only I could eat something, I could regain a little strength and figure out something.*

I ventured inside a makeshift deli that I had spotted from the field and pleaded for food, but all I received in return were hostile stares and gestures. I walked a few blocks more into a neighborhood with apartment buildings. Several young women dressed in baggy army pants and bandanas patrolled the street. "What neighborhood are we in?" I asked one of them. She answered, "Brownsville. And you don't look like you belong here."

One of the young women took pity on me and arranged for me to have a meal in a cozy storefront African restaurant. My food was solemnly served to me on china plates. As soon as I finished eating, the girl who had served my food pointed me in a direction, and I took off.

It had become a sunny, beautiful Indian summer day, which contrasted with my inner storms.

Anxiety squeezed all of the oxygen out of my body. I felt as if I might be living my last few days on earth.

Serge dominated my thoughts as I randomly turned corners. I kept trying to conjure up some series of events in which I could forgive him and we could happily be together. I had passed through several neighborhoods when a chubby bleached blonde fortyish woman approached me on the sidewalk and interrupted my reverie, "Honey, you look kind of lost. Are you looking for the subway?"

I wept and sputtered that I had no place to go. "Don't you worry. I want you to come with me. I have an errand, but then I'll take you home, and you can go right to sleep." I was happy to have the company. Her errand turned out to be showing up at a mental health outpatient clinic for a group session and to receive medication.

During her group session, I waited outside along with a number of other patients at the clinic. I began obsessing over where I was going to sleep and how I was going to survive.

Some of the patients huddled together in twos, walked to the corner, and then returned. I realized they were trading prescription pills, and it occurred to me that one of them must have some Ativan, Valium perfected, my favorite pill. One young woman did, but I didn't have the six dollars she wanted for three pills.

I searched through my purse for something of value. All I could find were my new glasses with a flattering pale lavender and silver wire designer frame that had been a gift from one of my uncles. Although legally blind without glasses, I reasoned that I still had my contact lenses and my prescription sunglasses.

I traded the $400 glasses for three Ativan pills, three anxiety erasers.

The young woman assured me that she was in front of the clinic almost every morning and would hold onto the glasses for a few days to exchange them back to me for the money.

Through the glass in the storefront, I glimpsed a doctor approaching the reception desk. I suspected he was a CIA plant ready to haul me inside, so I walked away without saying good-bye to my Good Samaritan.

A couple of neighborhoods later, a preppy looking young Black guy driving a convertible spotted me trudging along and offered me a ride back to Manhattan. I told him I was having terrible luck, and he produced some white powder in foil. Assuming it was speed, I sniffed it, happy for the boost. When we crossed the bridge into Manhattan, warmth and calm enveloped me as if I were taking a warm bath.

Before exiting the car, I remarked, "I've never had speed like this before. This is different."

My ride chuckled, "You thought I gave you speed. You're something else. I don't mess with that shit. That was heroin. Take it easy."

Later, I threw up from the heroin. I had no plan and no destination, but I still had enough Ativan to last me the day.

It was as if I were having a nightmare, but I wasn't. I was living one.

I had begun an affair with a stranger who was obviously spaced out on acid and to whom I was nothing but a warm body, an object.

I had stepped into a car with characters straight out of a dystopian horror film, and it had all seemed normal to me. What should have sent me running to safety, instead, intrigued me.

I felt as if I were jumping out of my own skin and was desperately longing to make that feeling stop. I wasn't thinking of anything but surviving the next few minutes.

The non-stop panic, alienation, and confusion, the racing thoughts, the disorientation—the mania was extremely painful. Any substance that would subdue the hysteria for a while seemed to be worth it.

CHAPTER 19

Streets of Manhattan

October 1988

Deep into the night, I could not stop shivering despite my layers of clothing. Homeless and dragging my possessions around in a cardboard box, it was impossible to ignore that something was horribly wrong, but I had no idea how to fix it. I wondered if my fate could be retribution for something terrible I had done in a past life.

I was supposed to be 3,000 miles away in Long Beach, California finishing my senior year in college and working as the entertainment editor on Cal State Long Beach's newspaper, *The Daily 49'er*. Mentally and physically, I was thousands of miles away from my former life as a coed, but I had no time for reflection because surviving on the streets kept me very busy.

I gravitated toward hospital waiting rooms for shelter and blended in with all of the others who endlessly waited in the identical rows of joined hard plastic chairs. When my face became familiar, I would get kicked out and begin the search for a new place to sleep.

During the day, I wandered around the city and occasionally took naps in neighborhood parks. I was living my life like the silver ball in a pinball machine that gets pushed from one random spot to another.

I was living my life like the silver ball in a pinball machine that gets pushed from one random spot to another.

Technically, I was clean. Running out of money had ended my weed smoking and tranquilizer popping. But I still craved them.

One night, too broke for subway tokens, I walked for over an hour, wind piercing through my cotton clothing and through my skin, to a drug rehab program.

In the black of night, I entered a waiting room overflowing with addicts, most of them bony and younger than thirty. I found a seat, grateful to be off my feet and in a warm room. Many of those waiting had fallen asleep in their seats while their heads hung awkwardly to their sides or backs.

The guy next to me tapped his feet, his hands, and his head as if in response to an irresistible beat. We began talking. He told me his nickname was China White in honor of his favorite brand of heroin. China had olive skin and dark, wavy shoulder-length hair. His slender, faintly muscular frame was clad in skin-tight jeans, a sleek pullover sweater, a black wool blazer, and pricey black cowboy boots.

"Are you trying to get into rehab?"

"No. I love heroin and I love using it. I've been using it since I was 16 years old. The only reason I'm here tonight is that a vein collapsed in my wife's arm, and I'm waiting for her."

Eventually, they released his wife, a young, frail blonde. Once China left, I had no one to talk to. Some dorky young guy whose drug of choice must have been Twinkies kept trying to get me to take a walk with him.

Sleep eluded me. I kept picturing Serge and wishing he was there with me. I had never seen him do drugs, but it was obvious he used something more than acid. I suspected he had friends all over the city, and I approached a group of sinister-looking guys to try to get them to reveal Serge's whereabouts. They didn't know what I was talking about, but I reasoned I hadn't found the right people yet.

The next morning a counselor informed me that the waiting list for rehab was several weeks. Something inside me snapped. I couldn't last another night on the streets.

I walked into a nearby shelter referral center. Once I started talking with the woman who assigned lodging, I began to cry and couldn't stop. I tried to explain my predicament, but desolation choked me. The woman wrote something down. She handed me an envelope and a subway token and said, "It's going to be OK. Take this envelope to the address I wrote on the outside of it."

It felt strange to ride the subway, especially for three stops. No longer crying, I presented the envelope to the shelter's receptionist. After a brief wait, I was instructed to take the elevator to the top floor to meet with Linda.

Linda's straight brown hair ended where her waist would have been had her fifty extra pounds not blurred her figure and her features. She bombarded me with questions regarding my family and background. Finally, I said, "I have to take a nap before I can answer any more questions. Could I lie down on that couch over there?"

When I awoke, Linda seemed upbeat, "I have someplace for you to go. Somebody you need to meet. I'm going to drive you there myself."

CHAPTER 20

ADHD, ADD, and Creativity

ADHD (attention deficit and hyperactivity disorder) and ADD (attention deficit disorder) are on a continuum. Earning a teaching credential and giving birth to two highly kinesthetic children prompted me to read a variety of books and articles about ADD.

Kinesthetic learner

If you tend to think in motion, you are probably a kinesthetic learner. A kinesthetic learner does not necessarily have ADD but simply requires more movement during the learning process.

In college, I eventually figured out that I needed to sit in front and take notes in order to follow along. Often, I can't read my notes, because of my sloppy left-handed handwriting. But if

I don't take notes, I can't understand what's going on. I space out, and the professor's voice fades into white noise.

My ideas for short stories, fiction, or articles generally come to me while I am moving—doing housework, taking a walk, or exercising.

Divergent thinking

Some experts debate whether you could have both bipolar depression and ADD or ADHD. In order to be highly creative, your brain has to be able to jump around and make unlikely connections.

Creativity is associated with divergent thinking, the process of creating many unique solutions to solve a problem. It is often described as spontaneous and free-flowing.

Convergent thinking

Whereas, convergent thinking relies heavily on logic. It's systematic and uses logical steps to figure out the single best solution.

Three components of creative thinking

"Three aspects of creative cognition are divergent thinking, conceptual expansion, and overcoming knowledge constraints. Divergent thinking, or the ability to think of many ideas from a single starting point, is a critical part of creative thinking," according to a 2019 *Scientific American* article, "The Creativity of ADHD: More insights on a positive side of a "disorder."

Previous research has established that individuals with ADHD are exceptionally good at divergent thinking tasks, such as creating recipes, writing songs, and brainstorming new features for appliances. "Together with previous research, these new findings link ADHD to all three elements of the creative cognition trio," according to the same May 2019 *Scientific American* article.

Left-handedness and ADD

Ten percent of the population is predominantly left-handed, and the wiring of left-handed brains differs somewhat from right-handed brains. "Left-handed students had a probability of suffering from ADHD 2.88 times greater than right-handers," according to a study published in June 2017 *Research in Developmental Disabilities*.

Left-handedness and mood disorders

Research also reveals that left-handed people are also more prone to mood disorders and schizophrenia.

CHAPTER 21

How Can Setting Goals Help You Focus?

Breaking down large goals into daily, weekly, and monthly goals enables me to achieve those large goals. Setting goals also decreases my anxiety and helps me focus.

Goal-setting has become one of my "anti-depressants." Outside of those goals related to my full-time job, the goals I set mainly have to do with writing and maintaining healthy habits. One of my weekly goals is to exercise five times during the week for an average of 45 minutes, including two resistance sessions.

Here are some benefits I get from setting goals:

1. **Focus on what's important.** The fear of forgetting makes me anxious. Even though I use a planner, a calendar,

my phone calendar, and notes on my wrist, I still forget important things once in a while.

Writing down daily goals helps me to remember appointments and due dates. When I glance at my daily list, it also helps chase away distracting thoughts.

2. **Focus on the solution.** Setting a goal, no matter how small, that takes me toward fixing or resolving a problem, helps shift my focus to what is in my control and away from feeling helpless.

3. **Simplify decision making.** For example, if I set a goal to get my chapter done by Friday, then I know I can't watch TV or do an Open Mic until it is done.

4. **Motivation**. It might sound silly, but it's fun to beat a deadline. Deadlines motivate me as well as energize me.

5. **Sense of purpose**. Thinking about what's important to me, making goals that reflect my values, and taking steps toward accomplishing what's important to me make me feel alive. Everything can be going great in my life, but if I'm not working towards a creative or personal goal in addition to the job-related ones, I feel a little down.

6. **Sense of possibility.** Breaking down larger goals into smaller achievable ones opens up the world of possibility and gives me something to imagine in the future—something to look forward to. In a word—empowering.

7. **Challenge**. Goals provide challenges, which energize me provided they're not overwhelming.

Find out more:

- "Effective Goal Setting Could Help People with Depression," Zawn Villines, January 5, 2017, GoodTherapy.org.

- "The Importance, Benefits, and Value of Goal Setting," Leslie Riopel, MSc., April 26, 2020, PositivePsychology. com.

PART THREE

Awareness

"For every one of us who succeeds, it's because there's some-body there to show you the way out."

–Oprah Winfrey

CHAPTER 22

Bellevue—Ward 19 North

October 1988

Minutes later, Linda parked her car in a vast lot not too far from some imposing buildings. We walked through the back door of one of the buildings into yet another waiting room. Linda told me to take a seat while she addressed somebody. The room was full of people. Most of them appeared downtrodden.

When Linda returned, she said, "Listen. You're going to have to stay here a few days until we can find a better place for you." I looked around and panicked, "What if I don't like it here?"

She patted me on the back and said, "Don't worry. It's only for a short time." Then she briskly walked out of the facility.

It occurred to me I had no way of getting back the remnants of my wardrobe I had surrendered to the shelter's reception desk. I headed to the service window where Linda had been talking to someone. "Where am I?"

"Bellevue Hospital. This is the psychiatric emergency room," a middle-aged woman answered. She looked as if she would be headed to choir practice after work.

Her answer made me feel as if I had been punched in the stomach. My enemies had plotted against me and won. My scream emerged as a croak, "I don't belong here. How do I get out of here?"

Matter-of-factly, she responded, "You can't leave until you've met with a doctor who will evaluate you."

"Well then let me get it over with. Where's the doctor?"

She raised her eyebrows and said sympathetically, "I'm afraid you're going to have to wait."

"How long?"

"It's hard to say. Hopefully, not more than a few hours. If you're hungry, don't worry. Dinner will be served any minute," she said and returned to her paperwork.

Sadness consumed me as I realized I had nowhere else to go. My weeks on the streets had zapped my energy and my spirit. A fellow waiting room occupant, an attractive thirty-something man whose skin had turned golden reddish-brown from the sun, interrupted my reverie, "Not the best place to be on a Friday night, huh?"

I answered, "I'd rather be anywhere than here."

Food trays arrived. I had not eaten in one or two days. The overcooked green beans, instant mashed potatoes, and rubbery boiled chicken made my mouth water. As we ate, Suntanned told me that he'd take me to a cheap motel when we were both released and that he'd take care of me.

Later that night, I met with a doctor and ended up screaming.

Shortly thereafter, A nurse wheeled in stretchers for those of us still waiting in the emergency room.

I woke up the next morning to a nurse signaling an orderly to move me to Ward 19 North. I asked the orderly which ward awaited Suntanned who was still asleep. He said he was not sure, probably the prison ward.

In the emergency room, only a security guard and a set of double doors had separated me from freedom. My new ward was 19 floors up and behind two sets of locked steel doors.

It only took a number of days for antipsychotic medications to rid me of my disabling symptoms, but Bellevue refused to discharge me because I didn't have a place to live. I desperately wanted to get a job and return to college, but the hospital's social worker shot down my plan. Her words stung, "Seven hospitalizations in eight years. Don't you think it's time to try something else?"

Before I could answer, she added, "You're 26—not that young anymore. Do you want to spend the rest of your life in and out of institutions?"

"Something else" turned out to be going on disability which would make me eligible for supervised living and health insurance.

During my three-month stay, I met with psychiatrists, some of them resident doctors in training, who listened to me. I realized that Ativan and Dalmane and similar medication had kept me from tuning into my shifts in behavior when the changes were subtle enough to arrest without progressing to mania.

Several weeks into my stay, I met with the supervising psychiatrist to request a change in my medication and she said, "If you can sleep through the night, I will take you off of everything, but your mood stabilizer."

True to her word, several days later, she did.

Because I had been a binge drug user, putting down drugs was not as hard for me as it is for some. Being in Bellevue for a prolonged time and reflecting upon the dangerous situations I had placed myself in convinced me that I risked my mental health by using.

However, I had zero understanding of addiction. I didn't realize that food had become my replacement tranquilizer.

By day, I attended ADEPT, Bellevue's therapeutic program that prepared outpatients to reenter society via occupational therapy, group therapy, and vocational counseling. I worked in one of the hospital's small cafeterias and eventually transferred to one of the gargantuan hospital's offices to perform basic secretarial duties. The routine and the opportunity to be productive agreed with me.

By night, I lived in an apartment program with other outpatients. Awkward.

Eventually, the ADEPT program graduated me to a software applications training program. The directors of ADEPT believed their graduates needed to earn a livable wage. The skills I acquired kept me from having to juggle two low-paying jobs and only be able to afford to rent space on someone's couch.

CHAPTER 23

Therapy

1989, New York City

Because the social workers at Bellevue and the apartment program had, on my behalf, gone through the bureaucratic nightmare of getting me temporary disability, I had health insurance for the first time since I was 19 years old.

This meant that, at 27, I could finally meet with a therapist. I began meeting weekly with Sarah. Sarah had a master's degree in clinical psychology and was working on her PhD at a teaching clinic in the Park Slope neighborhood of Brooklyn, which was walking distance from my apartment. She was in her forties, and therapy was a second career for her.

With Sarah, I opened up like an artichoke dipped in boiling water. Feeling so at ease with Sarah made me realize how guarded I had felt before. It had been so much hard work to make myself understood, and I had become sensitive about being judged. With Sarah, it didn't feel like work at all. She understood even my sentence fragments. When I was tired, I could be silent for a couple of minutes and simply be at ease.

In the womb of her tiny office, I could discuss anything with Sarah, even rape. I told her about the talk show I had recently watched in which rape victims had discussed how therapy was a crucial part of the process of healing from the trauma of rape. The show had made me reflect on how atypical my own experience had been.

I confessed, "I've been raped five different times, four of them during manic episodes, yet none of the rapes truly registered, because I was manic at the time. The rapes blended in with all of the chaos."

"When you say they didn't register, can you explain?" With Sarah, I felt the energy of someone intently listening to me and trying to connect. Time slowed down.

"I mean that rape, as terrifying as it was… It was not the worst thing I experienced. Those rapes were not the most awful things that happened to me." The conviction with which I had said that surprised me.

"What do you feel when you remember being raped?"

"Disgust that my impaired judgment put me in situations that made me vulnerable. That those rapes never would have happened had I not been manic. That I came close to being killed," I said and then sighed.

"Ironically, the rape that fills me with the most horror was an acquaintance rape, and that is the one during which I was not manic."

"What was more awful than being raped and almost killed?" Sarah asked softly.

"Being beaten up as a child," just saying those words made scenes flash through my mind.

"And also, I think it would be hard for someone to understand who hasn't been manic, but the opportunities I lost haunt me too."

My childhood trauma began when I was three or four years old. It took 23 years for me to work with a therapist, a gifted one at that, but I did finally get help. Not everyone is as fortunate.

I clung to the regularity of my therapy sessions like a skydiver clings to a parachute. In the midst of one of our sessions, I was surprised to discover that I often heard my father's voice in my head telling me how worthless I was.

"All those years we lived together, I blocked out all the disparaging things he said to me."

I pictured myself as a teenager forcing my mind to go elsewhere as he raged and often shook me and slammed my head into the wall. Snippets of scenes flashed through my mind along with a soundtrack of his oft-repeated put-downs.

"You're a slut."

"Your blood is tainted." (My father consistently brought to my attention that the genes I had inherited from my mother's mother doomed me as inferior.)

"You will never amount to anything. You're going to end up working at McDonald's."

Until that moment in Sarah's office, I had not realized these toxic put-downs my father had screamed at me during his frequent rages had been repeating themselves in my thoughts. This negative self-talk had become completely ingrained. It had become automatic thinking.

"It's not like I even believed him. When he lost it, he usually didn't make sense."

"Intellectually, you didn't believe him, but emotionally you did. You thought you were blocking his hurtful remarks out, but what you really did was bury them. And now they are coming to the surface."

Something still bothered me though. "But what I don't get is that it's not as if I lived through a war or a famine. I never went through a concentration camp or anything like that. Tons of people in the Third World are starving to death, and they're not depressed."

"Your father's abuse affected you. You are who you are. Everyone is different. Different people are affected by different things. Don't minimize the effect it had on you."

Sarah got me to acknowledge the abuse and to recognize the undercurrent of negative self-talk. She taught me how to shift away from the negative self-talk and combat the depression when it cropped up.

Looking back, many years later, do I think my father believed any of what he said? Not really. He disconnected when he raged. It was as if he had emotional blackouts akin to what happens to someone who has had way too much to drink. No true memory of what happened during the rage existed, just a vague recollection that he had gotten "upset." He has never acknowledged the six years of random beatings, destruction of property sessions, and twisted degradation.

My work with Sarah also helped me to let go of trying to answer why my father raged and to put his violence in context with all the good things he had done as a parent. Mainly, although he was not around much, he left me in good hands, whether it was neighborhood parents, his girlfriends, or family friends. He also enrolled me in solid public schools.

By my late twenties, I realized my father had done the best job he knew how with me and that he was incapable of acknowledging his violent and cruel behavior.

CHAPTER 24

Sleeping With the Enemy

1990

"Catherine?"

While navigating the crowded sidewalk, I heard my name being called before being able to figure out which hurried New Yorker had said it. Because few people knew me by that name, it couldn't be a case of mistaken identity.

A tall, slender twenty-something Asian-American man pulled away from the crowd, and I recognized him as my high school classmate Ben. We had been in the same honors classes in high school, and by senior year the calculus class had whittled down to about 15 students.

Ben had graduated from an Ivy League school and had become an architect. I was horribly impressed. I was so ashamed of my post-high school record that I simply mumbled I was working as an administrative assistant. (I had been thrilled to get a full-time job working for a non-profit arts organization in April, but compared to Ben's accomplishments, I felt like a loser.)

The Whitney Museum used to be located on the Upper East Side and within a half-hour walk from where I shared a one-bedroom apartment with a roommate in 1990 and 1991. I loved being in the proximity of a variety of museums. One winter evening, I had plans to meet Leslie, a friend from my software training program, after work at The Whitney. The night before, I had invited Ben to join us.

As we wandered around the museum, occasionally a piece of art would take my breath away with what it had captured, and I would have to look at it from different distances to fully appreciate it. The third time I did this, Ben looked at me as if I were a tacky tourist. For someone who made a living designing buildings, I was surprised Ben didn't have more to say about the paintings and other works of art on display.

While Ben was in the restroom, my friend Leslie whispered into my ear, "He seems kind of cold."

Ben and I had been hanging out here and there for a couple of months by the time he and I met for dinner in Chinatown.

When the bill came, I said, "Let's split it." Ben gave me that look to which I was becoming accustomed. It was between an almost laugh and a smirk.

What possessed me to follow him home after our dinner in Chinatown? I wasn't attracted to him. I never had been.

Was I that lonely? No. It was more like masochism. Like picking at a wound. Like I had a need to be degraded, and he fulfilled it.

The pain was palpable. Some part of me also knew that by sleeping with him I would get rid of him. He didn't really like me, but he did like looking down at me. He had tentatively pursued me for a couple of years in high school. Sleeping with him would satisfy his curiosity, and my lack of passion was bound to be a turnoff.

I woke up twisted in Ben's sheets on his twin bed. Once fully awake, that dreaded knot in my chest returned together with a mildly nauseous feeling in my gut. I became self-conscious of my face. I felt pale and as if my face had frozen. When moderately depressed, time slowed down, and I became overly aware of my body in the space it occupied.

Conveniently, Ben's apartment on the edge of Brooklyn was not far from Sarah's office. We had an appointment that Saturday morning.

As soon as I entered her office, I could tell she noticed something was wrong because she didn't say anything. Usually, we exchanged some pleasantries before our session, but that morning she was silent as we both took our seats.

"I just slept with someone I don't even like," I uttered. My words surprised me. The incident still seemed unreal.

"Oh, Sasha," Sarah said.

Verbalizing what I had experienced helped somewhat. After all the years of not being listened to about the abuse by relatives and then not being listened to by mental health professionals during my first eight years in treatment, having someone truly listen to me, recognize my strengths and my healthy parts, and believe in my future helped me achieve a critical turning point.

In the early 1990s, PTSD was generally only thought to relate to veterans, and I was never formally diagnosed with it. Depression related to PMS and PTSD is what I was going through as a teenager, and, at some point, I crossed the line into bipolar.

Was it smoking weed at 19 that took me over the edge? I will never know. There is an abundance of compelling research, which is reviewed in former *New York Times* reporter Alex Berenson's 2019 book *Tell Your Children: The Truth About Marijuana, Mental Illness, and Violence* as to the danger of using marijuana before the age of 25, particularly if there is any family history of schizophrenia or bipolar disorder.

To this day, I occasionally experience flashbacks of the abuse, but thanks to working with Sarah, I consider myself cured of PTSD because I no longer relive the episodes nor re-experience the trauma. The flashbacks go through my mind like any other memory. I no longer experience the episodes in nightmares either. That is significant because the nightmares used to disrupt my sleep, which led to depressive episodes.

My therapy with Sarah lasted one and a half years and ended when I left New York in late July of 1991.

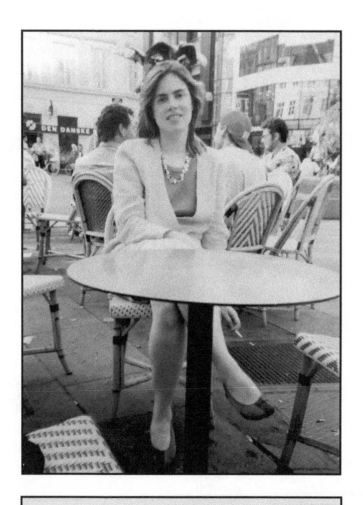

Copenhagen, Summer of '91. Before heading
back to college, I visited Scandinavia.

CHAPTER 25

Lasting Lessons From a Therapist

During my late twenties, my therapist, Sarah, taught me the tools I use to this day to combat anxiety and depression.

1. Treat yourself as if you were your own child. You wouldn't put down your child or say mean things to them. You would be gentle and loving.

2. When negative thinking or panic starts to build, focus on what you do have. Take yourself into the present by mentally making a quick gratitude list, such as...

   "Today I have a job. Today I have a place to live. Last night I slept for seven and a half hours."

3. Remind yourself that, although you are in some degree of pain, you are functioning. Mentally list the things you take for granted that you are accomplishing despite the lousy way you feel.

4. Why am I still stuck in low self-esteem? "You're used to it. Just like a pair of ripped, faded jeans are comfortable and hard to get rid of."

5. With regards to 12-step programs, take them cafeteria-style. Take what you like and leave the rest. (She wasn't suggesting you do sobriety part of the way, she was referring to such things as attending certain meetings, whether or not a certain sponsor's rules made sense for you, and that, at the time, most 12-step programs were highly skeptical of any medication for depression or bipolar disorder.)

CHAPTER 26

Final Semester

Fall 1991

There was a several week gap between when my job in Manhattan ended and when the fall semester began, and I used it to visit family and friends in Scandinavia.

At the age of 29, I returned to Cal State Long Beach. It was my last chance to get a degree with a major in journalism, my sixth major, because I had flunked the Law of Mass Communication twice and had to receive medical accommodation to attempt the class for the third and final time.

Writing journalism articles, I aced. Memorizing the details of case law, I floundered.

I loved everything about Cal State Long Beach. Students of all ages and backgrounds. Exchange students. A Music Listening Lounge. A Student Union that included a swimming pool, a bowling alley, and a room full of pinball machines.

Vendors selling cool, cheap clothes and more outside the bookstore.

Walking through the crowded, large campus gave me the same charge as walking the streets of Manhattan. But by midterms, the campus had become a blur. I felt nothing, and I noticed nothing as I walked through the campus. Depression distorts your perceptions. I had lost my ability to register my surroundings or react to much of anything. My sense of taste had all but disappeared too.

The night of my Law of Mass Communication midterm, I reread the essay questions as if by reading them over and over, the answers would miraculously come to me.

My fate was floating away from me. I had no Plan B. If I didn't get my bachelor's degree, I had no vision of my future. When I tried to picture my future, it was as if I were watching a TV screen that had turned into static.

I had no job, no car, and no apartment to call my own. Beyond hopeless. I felt paralyzed. I imagined ceasing to exist. I would try to imagine scenarios of a possible way out of my dismal existence, and I could not. If I couldn't make it through college after all the years invested, then what would I be able to do? Work some minimum wage job that only paid for food and transportation and rely on my family to house me?

I had thought that I was beyond the flashbacks I had worked through with Sarah in New York, but living with my grandmother that fall semester and interacting with my father brought them back.

I couldn't figure out a way out of my misery, and I couldn't answer the questions on the page. As if in a trance, I gathered my things and quietly exited the classroom.

As I shuffled through the hallway, my former Bellevue vocational counselor's words haunted me. He had strongly discouraged my returning to college to finish my degree. His preferred career for me had been a file clerk.

As I reached the exit to the building, I felt a tap on my shoulder. Startled, I turned around to face my 30-something professor. He had followed me out of the classroom.

With the zeal of a missionary, he talked to me about pressure and that it was something I could learn how to handle and not let it get to me.

I felt inadequate by comparison.

His words came through one by one and as if from a distance. By the time I comprehended one word, I had missed the next one. But his warmth and his concern somewhat penetrated through my haze.

When it was my turn to speak, all I could do was mumble about having studied for hours, but not being able to remember anything.

He reassured me that he could tell from my class participation that I knew the material, and he recommended using bullets to list key points in response to the test questions.

I slowly walked back into the classroom to face my adversary, a pale blue exam booklet. I outlined whatever I could, which was much easier than trying to form cohesive paragraphs.

Somehow, I passed the midterm, which eased my anxiety a bit.

A few days later, I had an appointment with a campus counselor. I had made the appointment at the beginning of the semester as a precaution. It would have been completely beyond me to make that appointment once the fog had descended.

I became much quieter when depressed. But unless you knew me extremely well, you would not notice anything amiss, because, around others, I slipped into my public persona.

The gray-haired counselor had a gentle voice. He reminded me of an elementary school teacher.

I could hear my own voice as I spoke. It sounded faint. I felt pathetic as I tried to explain that although I was studying for hours every day, nothing was sticking. When it came to exams, I couldn't connect anything.

The counselor looked so alive. I felt half dead.

He pointed out to me that I had been out of college three years and it took time to get back into the rhythm of academics and that studying was different than working.

I felt like such a loser. 12 years of college on the line. Why couldn't I coast through my last semester?

The counselor reviewed a typical day with me and came to the conclusion that I was overstudying.

What??? Overstudying! I had never heard of this. He continued to explain that studying for hours on end was actually counterproductive for some.

Suddenly I became alert as if the faint scent of hope had wafted into the room and refreshed me.

He handed me some stapled together papers that looked like a printout of a PowerPoint presentation. As he began flipping through the pages and pointing to various diagrams, his voice became more and more enthusiastic.

"Chunk out your time. Schedule study sessions throughout the day, and then break down your assignments into a list of tasks. After each study session, take a break. Do laundry, run an errand, read, take a walk. Anything different before your next study session."

Although skeptical, I took his advice. Miraculously, it worked. I did end up graduating that semester.

Years later, when I earned my teaching credential, I learned I had minor processing challenges and that was why I had excelled in some subjects and tanked in others.

CHAPTER 27

I'm Going to Marry Sasha

1992

During my final semester at Cal State Long Beach, I became acquainted with an outgoing and confident single man. Keith was only three years older than me and loved to play tennis. Actually, he was an accomplished tennis player who had chosen the variety of academic options a large state college had to offer over a tennis scholarship to a small liberal arts college.

Keith made me laugh—number one on my "list." And he nailed number two on my list—likes to play recreational sports.

We started dating the day I found out I would finally graduate from college. It was 10 days before New Year's Eve 1991.

For the first six months we dated, Keith would tell anyone in earshot, "I'm going to marry Sasha." I would laugh.

Whereas I tend to overthink almost everything, Keith was analytical, but not overly. His ability to quickly cut to the chase put me at ease as did his boyish quality and his infectious laugh. I could see why he had succeeded in sales. However, his territory had been all of California and Hawaii. He had grown tired of traveling and had returned to working in a more technical field that did not require travel.

Imagining a lifetime spent in Loserville engulfed me with feelings of despair every time I interviewed and didn't land yet another job. My temp agency was keeping me quite busy, but it wasn't the same as having a permanent job. It was a recession, but my negative self-image kept me from taking that into account. My job search was not focused. It didn't occur to me to look for jobs that involved business writing or to take advantage of Cal State Long Beach's career center.

Somehow, it did occur to me that I could have a future as a paralegal, and I enrolled in UCLA's Extended Education paralegal certificate program. I also managed to find an abysmal part-time job as a legal secretary in a family law practice. It marked the first time I had ever been treated with disdain on a job.

Just as my entire self-worth had been my grades, now my entire self-worth had become my work. Even though I had not had an episode of disabling depression, hypomania, or anything close for four and a half years, I struggled with lingering bouts of self-hatred.

CHAPTER 28

Manhattan Sidewalk Encounter

April 1993

Halfway through the paralegal certificate program I had been attending at UCLA, spring break beckoned. I also found myself in between temp assignments and decided to visit New York so I could clean out my storage unit there.

Once in New York and away from Keith, I became ambivalent about our relationship. As much fun as we usually had together, as much as I desperately wanted my own family, there was one key issue that was a deal-breaker, but, at the time, I didn't know myself well enough to know this.

As someone who used food to soothe, I wasn't in touch with many of my feelings. I had no understanding of addiction. New York Super Fudge Chunk is not nearly as deadly as heroin, but consuming mass quantities of it has a similar numbing effect. Over time, compulsive overeating causes more and more emotional damage in addition to making you overweight.

Back then, I thought an addict was someone who abused drugs or alcohol to the point that they ended up in prison, dead, or on Skid Row. I didn't think of overeating, gambling, compulsive spending, or compulsive relationships as variations on the theme of addiction.

Having cleaned out my storage unit, I felt free to roam around Manhattan my last few days in New York City and absorb the energy its infinite sidewalk scenes offered.

While using a payphone at the corner of 64th Street and First Avenue, I glimpsed a man out of the corner of my eye. In between my placing phone calls, he approached me. He asked me something about one of the shops in the neighborhood. His accent sounded German or Eastern European. Within a minute of talking with him, I realized he, Ingo, bore an uncanny resemblance to my favorite rock star, and I was intrigued. He was the same height and build. His hair was cut in the same loosely layered, just-past-chin-length style. However, he looked at least five years younger, and his hair was closer to curly than wavy.

He offered me one of his Dunhill Mild cigarettes, my favorite brand, although I hardly ever splurged for them. I tried to answer his question, "I'm not sure. The shops in the neighborhood have changed a little in the last two years. I used to live right up the block, but now I am visiting. I live in California."

"I live uptown. I'm an artist, but I do many small jobs. I probably make a sign for that store there, see?" He pointed to a small shop a few feet away.

He quickly, yet subtly shifted his weight from one foot to another. His restlessness was contagious. When he gestured, he kept his hands close to his body. We had been chatting for a few minutes when he interrupted. "What are you doing right now?"

"I was trying to reach a friend to make plans later, but couldn't get a hold of anyone. I'm going to walk back to my hotel."

"I'll walk you."

His offer made me light-headed, and I struggled to speak coherently. "It's over twenty blocks, but I love to walk, especially around the city."

"Me too," he pointed to his camera, "I always take my camera. New York is something. You never know what you see. It's just a hobby, but the photos give me ideas for my paintings."

As soon as we were seated and talking back in my hotel room, I noticed he had a slightly rebellious, slightly arrogant look. He dressed simply, but stylishly, and he immediately stood out as a European. He looked like the type I always imagined as my male counterpart, and, even better, he was an artist who oozed creativity.

I hadn't slept with a stranger in five years, but Ingo didn't feel like a stranger. He had emerged from one of my dreams.

"What's in your shopping bag?"

I showed him the black slingbacks I had purchased earlier that day. Their patent leather tips made them just glamorous enough for evening.

He held up one of the shoes and examined it from different angles as if it were a work of art. "Why don't you wear them, and change into something black to go along with the shoes."

Rummaging through my suitcase, I found a black knit sheath dress and black tights that had flowers patterned into their fishnet design. When I emerged from the bathroom clad in black, Ingo appeared subdued. He looked me over and then sat down in the chair and said, "Nice. Keep moving. I want to watch you."

Ingo's end of the conversation became mostly monosyllabic. I unpacked my reclaimed boom box, popped in a cassette salvaged from my storage unit, and began to sway to the music. After about twenty minutes, I strutted across the large room to where Ingo sat and asked him if he liked my new shoes.

"They're perfect for cocktail parties and sex," he answered.

I laughed.

He stood up. I took his arm and coerced him into twirling me. I kept twirling, and we eventually ended up fully clothed and tangled on the bed. After a few minutes of brushing up against each other, I was moaning.

The safest sex I had ever had. I was surprised that my body had responded so easily. It reminded me of my early days in college when I had been a virgin and kissing a date could give me goosebumps.

Later that evening, I caressed his body as if he were a piece of sculpture my hands were trying to memorize. When he was no longer capable of standing, we ended up on the floor.

While being entwined with Ingo, the waves of pleasure became more and more intense. When I closed my eyes, I saw silver, white, and lavender sparks of light exploding.

After we'd caught our breath, he became introspective and told me about his life, mainly how he had struggled to establish himself as an artist and what he had gone through to get to the United States. Comforted by the realization that I had been destined to break up with Keith and meet Ingo, I drifted into a light sleep while still on the floor.

Sometime during the wee hours, Ingo took a long, steamy shower in the bathroom that looked as if it had been around since the 1940s. He exited the bathroom with a towel wrapped around his waist. Just waking up from a catnap, I admired his toned body. His torso could have been a centerfold.

He seemed to walk more loosely. His hair looked softer, less curly, and his Eastern European accent softened. He impressed me by boiling water for tea in a metal canister, as I didn't have a kettle.

Ingo donned my Cal State Long Beach sweatshirt, and we ventured out amidst the giant billboards, marquees, and brightly lit stores to a Howard Johnson's in the Times Square district. If I squinted, it felt as if we were in a psychedelic funhouse. We sat in a booth overlooking the harsh lights, and I experienced déjà vu.

Greasy chicken wings and bland breaded food seemed charming in Ingo's company. In his presence, I felt relaxed and charged up at the same time. We didn't talk much, but we communicated a lifetime when we looked into each other's eyes.

The next morning, I was in a haze, so sleepy it was as if I were mildly stoned. Ingo's face approached a smirk, amused at the extent of my passion as we made love.

Ingo, watching me struggling to pack all of my things into my suitcase, laughed at me and muttered, "Fellini movie." I was too dazed to realize that I had been insulted.

Once all of my belongings were packed, Ingo said, "I want you to see my apartment before you leave." I was relieved to not have to say good-bye yet. I silently followed Ingo into the subway memorizing the almost mechanical way he walked and how he looked in a perfectly cut black leather jacket, black jeans, and sexy shoes. Underground, everything appeared vivid and to move slightly in slow motion. Colors looked brighter. The resolution had been heightened. The passengers' features popped out at me. The subway felt like an amusement park ride. Ingo even looked cool grasping the subway pole.

When we emerged above ground Ingo said, "See the border. I'm right on the border." He was referring to the border of Spanish Harlem. He lived in the East 90s. His apartment was on the ground floor of a sooty four-story walk-up. Its facade was deceptive. Inside his apartment, the kitchen counters were meticulously tiled in shiny square-inch black tile. One long counter accommodated three stools. I was so surprised by the sight of his kitchen that I couldn't stop admiring it.

"I did all the work here. It didn't look like this when I moved in," Ingo said as he opened one of the pale beige wood cabinets to put away some mugs that had been drying next to the stainless-steel sink.

Ingo gave me a quick tour of the rest of the apartment. Its only flaw was that the rooms were connected to each other in railroad car fashion. When we walked through one bedroom to get to the other bedroom, Ingo said, "I have a roommate, but he's at work."

Light hardwood floors, high ceilings, moldings, and fresh paint made the apartment feel like an oasis from the grimy city. The apartment was so spotless and tastefully furnished for two bachelors, I almost questioned Ingo's sexuality. When we walked back into the living room, Ingo showed me some of his colorful, striking paintings.

His paintings spoke to me. They conveyed emotions, impressions, and scenarios. Part of me had hoped I would not like his work at all because it would have made it easier to forget about him. Instead, I fell in love with his artwork, which reminded me of two renowned abstract expressionist artists, Helen Frankenthaler and Richard Diebenkorn.

He showed me two similar small canvasses done predominantly in primary colors and told me he wanted me to buy one of them. I walked around the room looking at one of them and kept seeing different things from different angles and distances. From across the room, I saw seagulls flying across a crowded colorful summer beach scene. They appeared to be in motion. Closer up and from the side, I saw a distorted Renoir café scene, Renoir on acid.

He presented a price list from a past gallery showing and they listed at $595. He said, "I wouldn't want you to pay me that. I just want to show you what they are worth. Anything, just something, so you bought it. Twenty dollars is great." I handed him sixty dollars over his objections.

Surrounded by a bustling weekday lunch crowd, Ingo and I sat at a small table solemnly staring at each other. Between the bright, unnatural light emanating from the overabundance of track fluorescent lights and the all-white decor, the restaurant reminded me of an operating room. Ingo seemed nervous. He looked frail beneath his sun-tanned skin. I rearranged the artichokes in my enormous salad and broke the silence by babbling about looking forward to returning to California.

I could not stop talking. Associations and ideas built up momentum begging to be released like the steam forming from water boiling in a tea kettle.

The waiter hurriedly refilled my iced tea and I said, "But the bad thing is I'll never see you again."

"I'll come to visit you." He smiled warmly which made him look at least ten years younger.

I removed a lemon wedge from the edge of my tall glass and squeezed as much lemon juice as I could into my iced tea, stirred in some more Sweet-n-Low, and sipped my iced tea. "How will you know how to find me?"

He grinned, "I'll find you. Just dream about me. He put down his fork and motioned slightly with his arms and shoulders as if he were flying, "I'll fly out, and we can make love on the beach."

Visualizing such a scenario sent warm tingles up and down my torso. I pictured a photo of my favorite rock star, shirtless, lying sideways across a bed. He was alone in a barren room. He looked completely relaxed. The backs of his knees were bent against the edge of a stark white mattress. The photo, inset against a cloud-like wash of sky blue and white, made him look as if his spirit was preparing to fly away from his body. All the puzzle pieces magically came together. Ingo and I were about to embark on a mystical relationship.

Sensing that this might be the last time I would ever see Ingo in the flesh, I felt compelled to remove one of the two slender unisex silver chain bracelets I was wearing. His hand trembled when I placed one of them on his bony wrist. Its silver strands were entwined in an unusual geometric pattern, sort of fishtailed, but not exactly. "Now we're matching," I said.

After I paid the lunch bill, we picked up my suitcase from the hotel's front desk and headed toward Grand Central Station to catch a train. I planned to spend my last couple of days in New York with Aunt Leah. We killed time by sitting on my black hardback suitcase and listening to some musicians playing blues music in the main area of the station. It felt comfortable, but within half an hour it was time to board my train. Ingo walked me to the train. I turned to kiss him good-bye. He reluctantly kissed me and then pulled away and said, "You should never do that in public."

I laughed and waved my hand around, "We're beside train tracks. Everyone is hurrying around. No one noticed." He looked at me as if to say, *You are a silly girl,* and ever so slightly shrugged before whispering, "Good-bye."

Our encounter had left me euphoric. I reflected upon it while I hung out by myself in Aunt Leah's basement and boxed for shipment the few belongings that remained from my storage unit. I studied Ingo's painting and fantasized about watching him in the act of creating it. If I stared long enough at it, maybe I could communicate telepathically with him. Maybe we could even share an out-of-body experience. I didn't feel ready to be 3,000 miles away from him.

I dialed Ingo's number. When he picked up the phone, it was difficult to communicate. There were no gestures to help me interpret his limited vocabulary. I hung up feeling confused and as if I needed to see him once more before I left. I changed my reservation so I could stay five more days, which meant I would miss only one night of paralegal class.

Only one day's worth of Tegretol pills remained in my prescription bottle. I called my doctor in California who informed me that he could not write an out-of-state prescription and suggested I go to Bellevue's walk-in clinic. Bellevue's clinic seemed like one step from being locked up, so I decided to go without for the few extra days I'd be in New York.

The next day Aunt Leah watched me propping up Ingo's canvas and said, "Please tell me you bought it at a flea market, that you did not pay good money for it. That is one of the ugliest paintings I have ever seen. It looks like splattered paint."

We got into a senseless argument. I grabbed my purse and ran out the door without a jacket. I walked a mile to the train station shivering the entire way in the cool March air.

Sex with Strangers

Sex, a rush... extraordinary...
The most potent drug.

Warmth. Connection. Sleep.

Sex with strangers
Courting danger

So many years ago
Out of character

Impaired judgment
Thoughts rushing, popping, colliding
Excruciating pain

Fragmented memories
As if watching an art movie
Kaleidoscope

A Fix Like No Other

Anticipation

Connection

Warmth, touch, and hearts beating faster.
Sex

CHAPTER 29

Relapse

Summer 1993, New York City

I still did not think of myself as an addict as my usage was not as extreme as most other drug users. I knew I had behaved as a drug addict while manic, but I did not understand the dynamics of addiction. I did not realize that I simply traded my fixes while in remission. Instead of easing my anxiety with drugs, I used food and codependent relationships to deal with them while in remission, which was most of the time.

By July 1993 Ingo had drifted away, but I was still in New York City. I had traveled far from the land of remission. I don't usually frequent bars, especially by myself, but I was not myself.

I hate the way people behave while drunk, but bars and alcohol go together.

There were several bars within a four-block radius from my apartment. Alcohol had never been my drug of choice because being drunk felt like a complete loss of control. I had much preferred pills, because they eliminated my anxiety, yet left me feeling in control. But they were not around, and I was afraid of getting hooked on them again.

I drank just enough, two to four drinks, to have the courage to pick up men.

Sex with strangers became my solace. When out on the prowl, I often wore one of two outfits, a fitted rayon navy blue suit with a short skirt that could have been stolen from the set of a cheesy television drama or a gray cotton and lycra unitard with a dark gray suede shirt-jacket. The jacket had been in mint condition when I had found it neatly folded atop a box next to someone's trash bins.

There was something thrilling about walking into a new bar for the first time. I would scope out the jukebox and select as many good songs as possible, which always took a while. Guns and Roses' "Sweet Child of Mine," Supertramp's "The Logical Song," and The Rolling Stones, "Gimme Shelter" were some of my favorites. The songs were always cheaper when you paid for several of them at once. It was impossible to tell how many songs were cued up ahead of mine. The anticipation of waiting for my first song to play made the song sound even better once it did play.

After selecting my songs, I would scope out the single men on my way to an empty seat at the bar.

Breathe. Relax. Keep soaking it in... ran through my thoughts. Once I had my first drink in me that was easier to do. Gin and certain types of wine instantly gave me a headache. I didn't like the taste of beer. That left me with vodka and tonic, vodka and grapefruit juice, vodka and cranberry juice, or vodka and anything. My favorite vodka drink of all time was a Malibu Wave, which achieved its seafoam green color from a shot of Midori.

In Long Island City, there were no Malibu Waves and no Malibu guys.

One night, I woke up restless at 2:00 a.m. Having taken to sleeping in my clothes, I grabbed a jacket, my purse, and my Walkman and wandered out the door. The sky resembled infinite shades of gray and black. The sidewalks on my horizon reminded me of textbook illustrations of perspective.

I walked for miles enjoying the city still lifes—silent playgrounds, locked storefronts, and empty streets all lit by streetlamps.

The music sounded better against the absolute quiet. It blared through the speakers of my Walkman and straight into my soul. I believed the music's vibrations, particularly those from U2's "Achtung Baby" created a protective aura around me that kept anyone from harming me on my pre-dawn walks.

CHAPTER 30

Back Together

August 1993

One morning, I woke up with my heart in my stomach. Depressed. The mania had disappeared overnight, and suddenly I was cognizant of my recent behavior—horrified. Longing for Keith consumed me. I immediately called him and blurted, "I miss you."

"I miss you too. It is so good to hear your voice. It was as if you were another person."

"I can't believe this happened again."

Deep down I knew Keith was not right for me in one critical way, and that realization that I could not come to terms with, that fear of loss, had served as a catalyst in my relapse. Sometimes, right when I start to get depressed, I would see situations in my life in a harsh light. Sometimes that harsh light was more accurate than my day-to-day perceptions, and

142

sometimes my perceptions were distorted and inaccurate. I had survived my childhood by blocking out the abuse. In retrospect, it seemed as if I still compartmentalized negative treatment of me.

Sarah had pointed out that some people tend to return to what we are used to, what is familiar, even if what we are used to is not good for us.

Keith was my life raft. My comfort. My focusing agent. I trusted him. I trusted his innate goodness and his practical intelligence.

When I look back, I was terrified of being alone. I had no understanding of addiction and a modest understanding of bipolar disorder. However, I had been blessed with several advantages that I had not had before Bellevue:

- My willingness to put down addictive prescription benzodiazepines, despite that, with my diagnosis, those drugs were always only a phone call away.

- Sarah. The year and a half I had worked with her had brought some buried pain to the surface, given me an awareness of my negative self-talk, and given me some cognitive tools with which to combat the negative self-talk.

- A degree in journalism, which had taught me how to evaluate research and interview experts.

CHAPTER 31

Whether to Have Children

1995

Although I had wanted to become a mother since my brother had been an infant, I struggled with whether to try for a child when Keith and I married in 1995. Even though I had been stable for two years since my relapse and five years before it, I wondered if it was fair for me to bring a child into this world. Because there was no history of manic depression in my husband's family, I wasn't overly worried about my child's chance of inheriting the illness.

I was worried about my health. If I got sick, who would take care of my child? I wanted a guarantee that I'd never get sick again. There is no such thing.

My doctor at the time, Dr. Amber, helped me mull over the decision, and I realized I did have faith in myself and in my marriage. I reasoned that as long as I continued to make my health my priority and maintained a positive working relationship with a psychiatrist, there was no reason for me to ever become psychotic again. That's not to say I believed I'd never again struggle with depression or pre-manic symptoms, such as occasional obsessive-compulsive thoughts, but if those symptoms continued to be as subtle and infrequent as they had become, then I believed I could be a loving, nurturing mother.

Six months after getting married I began writing a novel. I had not written anything since my manic episode in the summer of 1988. Opportunities had presented themselves, but I had not at all been interested.

True writer's block is when you don't see yourself as a writer. The drive is not only gone, you can't remember that it existed. I had never discussed writing in therapy because I had completely blocked out my creative side.

Getting married made me feel as if I had a true home, my home. This sense of security enabled me to let down my guard enough to remember how much I loved to write. I began writing a novel based on the bond that developed between myself and Amy and my other close friend that first semester at Coracle. We were well-rounded, outgoing, and down-to-earth, but all three of us had felt like outsiders. None of us ended up graduating from Coracle.

1998

The novel ended up reading like a non-mystery Nancy Drew novel, and, by 1998, I had abandoned it and was writing comedic screenplays.

Pregnancy agreed with me. I slept close to nine hours a night and felt the calmest I ever have. Because of my history with miscarriages, and because I celebrated my 36th birthday shortly before getting pregnant with my son, I opted to stay off medication while pregnant. Dr. Amber supervised me through my pregnancy, and a high-risk ob-gyn treated me with progesterone during the first trimester to prevent another miscarriage.

Without the high-risk ob-gyn's detective work, deducing that the most likely reason for my recurrent miscarriages had been my body's inability to produce enough progesterone, I would never have given birth to my son. My progesterone level had tested borderline, and it had previously been ruled out as a cause, but my miscarriages had happened around 10 weeks, which is often the case when one's body doesn't produce enough progesterone to support a pregnancy. Progesterone is inexpensive, easy to self-administer by suppository, and only needed during the first trimester.

Although I had explained to my ob-gyn that I needed to exercise as an antidepressant, he had said with a smile, "You'll be fine walking. It's different when you're pregnant. No running. You can swim too."

I trusted him, and I listened to him. However, after the amnio, I had contractions and was on bed rest for approximately two weeks before returning to work. During those two weeks, I couldn't do pretty much anything, and I watched the 1998 US Open Tennis Championship all day. Patrick Rafter won for the second time.

Coincidentally, I had sat about 10 feet away from Patrick Rafter on practice courts at the former Volvo Los Angeles tournament and at the Indian Wells tournament. He served and volleyed a lot, which was fun to watch. I remembered that he had appeared more buff in person than on TV. After researching his character through varied newspaper and magazine accounts from Australia, the US, and England, I decided to name my son after him.

CHAPTER 32

Q&A Interview With Dr. Roger McIntyre

Bipolar Depression and "Addiction"—The Relationship

Roger McIntyre, PhD, Professor of Psychiatry and Pharmacology, University of Toronto, Director of Depression and Bipolar Support Alliance (DBSA)

Q: Considering drug/alcohol addiction, gambling, compulsive eating, and other compulsive behaviors, do you think most individuals diagnosed with bipolar disorder struggle with addiction?

A: We no longer use the word addiction. It is true that the majority of people who have bipolar disorder at some time in their life will be affected by an additional condition that reflects a disturbance in what we call reward behavior. This includes, but is not limited to, alcohol-related problems and/ or substance-related problems and/or obesity.

Q: Do the bipolar symptoms tend to drive the drug, alcohol, or food abuse?

A: There's no question that for some people, some of the symptoms are responsible for the misuse of excess food consumption and/or drug and alcohol misuse. However, it's not only the symptoms, but it's also part of the illness.

For example, as part of the illness, many people have problems with impulse control that relates to cognition and also difficulties with what we call reward behavior. Reward behavior is a vague term that generally refers to behaviors that might be excessive, which result in the overconsumption and the use of substances that are affecting reward aspects of the brain.

Q: How likely is it that the addiction will disappear once the mood swings are stabilized?

A: In many cases, drug and alcohol misuse, as well as chaotic eating, may improve as symptoms of mania or depression improve. HOWEVER, the great majority of people continue to have the foregoing problems even when symptoms are in full remission. This is why it's important to pay very close attention to this issue all the time.

Q: For individuals with a dual diagnosis, do they need treatment for addiction as well as bipolar depression?

A: Yes. It is essential that both conditions are treated at the same time. Active drug and alcohol addiction interfere with treatment.

Q: Does compulsive overeating interfere with bipolar treatment?

A: Certainly, obesity might affect response to some treatments. We know that obesity and bipolar disorder worsen depression and cognitive dysfunction. There is a suggestion that some medications for bipolar disorder might not be as reliably effective in people who are also affected by obesity.

Q: How might a ketogenic, keto, diet help with symptoms of bipolar depression?

A: We have no data on this at this time. This is an area that is being actively studied. For now, what's recommended is a balanced healthy diet.

Q: How can routines help someone manage bipolar, and can they improve cognitive function?

A: Proper sleep, structured day, good exercise, managing weight, minimizing alcohol consumption, avoiding cannabis, as well as avoiding medications that interfere with cognition prevent episodes of depression and mania and are the best ways to preserve and improve cognition in people who have bipolar disorder.

Q: Why is at least seven hours of sleep a night critical to someone with bipolar?

A: Every person is different and I would not say that seven hours is a must for every individual. It is true that most people in the population require approximately seven to eight hours of sleep.

The key thing is to achieve the number of hours of sleep that are normal for you. Secondly, make sure you have a regimen where you sleep and wake at about the same time every day. Thirdly, do what you can to reduce disruptions of your sleep by improving sleep hygiene (e.g. avoiding activating behaviors late at night, such as using devices).

CHAPTER 33

Routines Benefit Depression and Bipolar Depression

Role of circadian rhythms

The circadian rhythm is the 24-hour internal clock controlled by the hypothalamus (a region of the forebrain) that affects hormonal cycles, body temperature, and your sleep/wake cycle.

Ideally, your circadian rhythm should cycle between sleepiness and alertness at regular intervals throughout the day.

Bipolar disorder is closely linked with having a shaky circadian rhythm. Regular activity, routines, help counteract this. Routines, even simple ones, can promote regular sleep, improved mood, and increased productivity.

Meals at the same time

Research has shown that eating meals at the same time every day helps synchronize the circadian system.

Your body consists of complex systems and digesting food influences the circulatory system, endocrine system, and excretory system.

Sleep

Getting to bed and waking up at the same time, or close to it, every day and getting adequate sleep is critical for someone with bipolar depression. (This was not explained to me until my last hospitalization, years after diagnosis.)

When tempted to work into the wee hours, I remind myself that if I don't get enough sleep, my shaky circadian rhythm will disrupt my brain circuitry, which could lead to mania. Mania can lead to judgment so impaired I could inadvertently place myself in life-threatening circumstances.

IPSRT

Interpersonal and Social Rhythm Therapy (IPSRT) teaches individuals how to understand and work with their biological and social rhythms in order to improve their moods.

Research has shown that routines can benefit addiction and depression as wells as bipolar depression.

Benefits of routines

When you have routines in place, you know what to expect, it's easier to organize yourself around your routines, and it frees up your brain for higher-order skills, such as planning and imagining.

Routines make it easier to actively work toward counteracting negative thoughts and symptoms.

Find out more:

- Sasha Kildare, "Routine Maintenance: How Sticking to a Schedule Helps Maintain Balance," bp Magazine, Winter 2017. bphope.com.

- Ipsrt.org, Interpersonal Social Rhythm Therapy.

- Mariana Plata, MSc, "The Power of Routines in Your Mental Health," *Psychology Today,* PsychologyToday. com, October 4, 2018.

- Brain and Behavior Research Foundation, "Circadian Rhythms and Bipolar Disorder," BBRFoundation.org, April 9, 2019.

CHAPTER 34

Anxiety, Depression, and Low Self-Compassion— The Relationship

Anxiety, depression, and low self-compassion can interact, and sometimes it's hard to sort out how they influence each other.

Anxiety = What if? **Depression** = Why bother? **Low self-compassion** = I suck.

When I am experiencing major stress, I battle symptoms of what I call mild depression, but those symptoms more easily classify as anxiety and a lack of self-compassion.

Low self-compassion

Self-compassion means that you are kind to yourself and able to notice your thoughts and feelings in the present moment without judging yourself.

A lack of self-compassion is said to be characterized by:

• Feeling isolated

• Lack of mindfulness

• Harshly critical of oneself

• Inability to be kind to yourself

Most of the time I have learned to ignore the negative, internal dialogue that can emerge from my subconscious. Stepping back and becoming aware of this dynamic when it surfaces enables me to fight it and to make it disappear for a while— sometimes for a long while.

Symptoms of depression

Depression is a commonly used term, but clinical depression means you have symptoms that affect your daily functioning and last for at least two weeks. Not everyone who experiences depression experiences all of these symptoms, but common symptoms include:

• Changes in activity level

• Hopelessness or guilty thoughts

• Lack of interest in activities

• Losing your appetite or eating too much

• Loss of energy

- Physical aches and pains
- Sleeping too much or having difficulty getting to sleep
- Suicidal thoughts
- Trouble concentrating

Symptoms of anxiety

Anxiety is uncomfortable. It is categorized by non-stop fear or worry and one or more of the following symptoms:

- Feelings of apprehension or dread
- Feeling tense or jumpy
- Restlessness or irritability
- Anticipating the worst and being watchful for signs of danger

Anxiety often translates into physical symptoms:

- Diarrhea
- Fatigue and insomnia
- Headaches
- Needing to urinate more often
- Pounding or racing heart
- Shortness of breath
- Sweating
- Tremors or twitches
- Upset stomach

Feelings of apprehension or dread and a racing heart are the symptoms I experience.

Self-Compassion can Alleviate Anxiety and Depression

Research studies haven't been able to sort out exactly how effective self-compassion therapy is for alleviating chronic anxiety and depression.

Research psychologist and author Kristen Neff specializes in the study of self-compassion and describes its role in reducing anxiety and depression in *Greater Good Magazine,*

"When we soothe our agitated minds with self-compassion, we're better able to notice what's right as well as what's wrong, so that we can orient ourselves toward that which gives us joy."

Find out more:

- Kristen Neff, "Why Self-Compassions Trumps Self-Esteem," *Greater Good Magazine*, May 27, 2011.

- Amy Louise Finlay-Jones, "The relevance of self-compassion as an intervention target in mood and anxiety disorders: A narrative review based on an emotion regulation framework," *Clinical Psychologist 21* (2017) p. 90–103.

- Nicole Snaith et al., "Mindfulness, self-compassion, anxiety and depression measures in South Australian yoga participants: implications for designing a yoga inter-vention," *Complementary Therapies in Clinical Practice*, Volume 32, August 2018, p. 92-99.

- Alexander C. Wilson, et al., "Effectiveness of Self-Compassion Related Therapies: a Systematic Review and Meta-analysis." *Mindfulness* (2019) 10:979–995.

PART FOUR

Awakening

"It takes courage to change."

–Alexandra Ocasio Cortez

CHAPTER 35

Becoming a Mother... Grieving My Mother

January 1999

After I gave birth to my son, I cried for my mother.

During one of those sleep exhausted postpartum days, I remembered a conversation I had with Mor Mor about Dorothy, my godmother. I met Dorothy for the first time during my senior year of high school when I interviewed at Wellesley College and stayed with her and her family in Boston.

Although Dorothy was only in her early forties when I met her, she looked 20 years older. Many of her fingers were stumps. I found out later from another college friend of my mother's that she had set herself on fire in religious fervor and disfigured her hands.

Dorothy showed me around Boston and later that evening surprised me with a Degas poster I had admired. She was gentle and didn't say much. What she did say sounded slightly stilted. I also found out later that she took medication, lithium I believe.

Mor Mor had tried to prepare me, "You know Dorothy had a nervous breakdown right after college. She was newly married and ended up in the hospital for quite a long time. It was devastating. Dorothy told me that Cynthia was the only one of her friends that had come to visit her regularly in the hospital, and Dorothy could never forget how much that had come to mean to her at the time.

"After you were born, your mother chose Dorothy to be your godmother."

That memory flooded me with conflicting emotions— sorrow for having lost my mother and her tremendous spirit, comfort that my mother would have seen through my illness to the person within, and gratitude that Mor Mor had spent many years telling me stories about my mother. My mother's death had been such a tragedy that most of my relatives flinched whenever her name was mentioned.

Shortly before my son's birth, we bought a blonde wood minimalist style rocking chair that came with a footrest. Both pieces were upholstered in rugged pale blue fabric shot through with pastel peach thread, and we parked them near a floor-length window that had a southern exposure.

One morning shortly after Patrick's birth, I nursed him in the comfort of the rocking chair. Sunlight poured in through the window and soothed me, and I was overcome with memories of being in my mother's presence. It was as if giving birth to my son had brought my mother back to me.

As I held my son and gazed into his eyes, I was able to remember the maternal love that I had felt so strongly from my mother, such as when I had injured my shin not long before she died.

I sat trembling on my mother's lap trying to bury myself in her chest and arms. We were in the doctor's office. I had been climbing the monkey bars at nursery school, and a protruding nail had ripped apart my right calf near my shinbone. My mother had left work to fetch me.

Her soft voice sounded like gentle surf as she whispered in my ear, "When the doctor sews up your leg, it's going to hurt."

"I'm scared Mommy," I said as warm tears began to slide down my cheeks.

"Don't be scared. Don't cry. You're my brave little soldier."

"Maybe my leg will get all better by itself," I said.

"No, darling. It won't. Show the doctor how brave you can be. Then you and Mommy can go home."

After she died, I'd stare at my faded long scar, which resembled a seam coming undone, to prove to myself that she had existed.

My friends and relatives are amazed that I remember so many little things about my mother because I was only three years old when she died. Her death was such a shock to me, it seared those memories into my psyche. Also, she was such an amazing mother—creative, loving, and giving of herself.

Had my mother not died, I would not have spent most of my childhood getting beaten up, emotionally abused, and repeatedly having my head banged against a wall. It is possible that bipolar disorder would never have been triggered. It is impossible to know for sure.

Had I not been blessed with such a nurturing mother during those critical first three years of life, I might not have been able to untangle the web of bipolar disorder, addiction, and trauma.

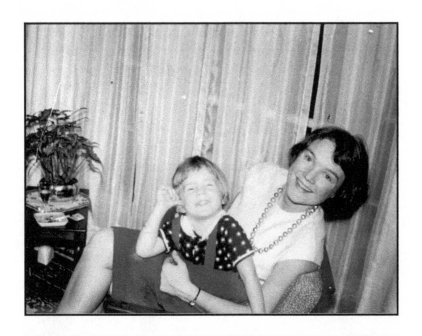

My mother and I on her 29th birthday four and a half
months before her fatal car accident.

CHAPTER 36

Postpartum

February 1999

I paced the short length of my tiny third-floor balcony as I smoked. Streetlights illuminated the deserted city street below.

A figure emerged clad in garments as blue-black as the sky. I glanced at my wristwatch. The time was 3:30 a.m. Blue Guy stared at me before sauntering down the block. He waved his arms in slow-motion like a balletic traffic cop. His signals jogged my memory. I took a deep drag of my cigarette as I thought of years past when I had not been watching from the safety of a balcony, but walking the streets at all hours of the night.

Eleven years past, during that hazy period right before Bellevue, another nightcrawler had interrupted my sojourn on the streets of Manhattan. He had insisted that I come home with him and his family. Technically homeless, I couldn't think of a reason not to follow him home. We had emerged from the subway into a neighborhood in which gang members patrolled the streets and directed traffic.

His "family" had lived in a sprawling basement apartment. They had offered me a bed in a room three lesbians shared, but when my newfound acquaintance had demanded I take a shower, I got scared and left. I had been bleeding heavily, unsure whether I had been miscarrying.

I guiltily lit up another cigarette knowing that its poisons filtered into my breast milk. I timed my one or two cigarettes a day to be after nursing and pumping. Pregnancy had kept me from nicotine. Sleep deprivation had brought back the cravings.

Right before my due date, I had opted to nurse, which meant I could not resume lithium until I was done nursing.

Coercing my body into producing enough milk to feed my newborn meant seven feedings a day, as many times pumping, and three doses of herbal tea that tasted like twig water. Every time I looked at the hospital-grade breast pump, I heard the fates laugh at me for going against medical advice, staying off medication to nurse my first-born.

The sleep interruption that resulted from the numerous feedings and pumping sessions sparked symptoms. I could not stop talking at times, and I could not sleep soundly.

Dr. Amber was furious with me, as I had gone against her medical advice, which had been not to nurse. To avoid nipple confusion, I was trying not to give my son a bottle for his first few weeks of life.

"Nipple confusion," Dr. Amber said exasperatedly, "You go straight to your pediatrician and your lactation consultant and tell them you are bipolar, and you must figure out a way you can sleep more than two hours at a time. If you have to go to the hospital, you won't do your son any good."

I had never seen Dr. Amber upset before. I trusted her and I respected her, so I took what she said to heart. She had always been positive and encouraging and had confided her own many-years struggle with infertility until, in her early forties, finally giving birth to a daughter.

Keith ended up giving our son a bottle in the morning, which allowed me to sleep for four hours straight. For the first several days, I didn't sleep much during the day when I napped, but I was terrified of becoming manic and having to abandon nursing. There was no going back to nursing once your milk supply had dried up.

Whenever our son napped during the day, I would lie in bed, darken the room as much as possible, play ocean sounds, and do breathing exercises. The breathing calmed me down and slowed me down by crowding out my anxious thoughts.

In addition to strolling with our son during the day, every evening, I forced myself to get out of the house and walk to Bluff Park, which overlooked the beach and was only a brisk ten-minute walk from our condo. Bluff Park was named after its rugged cliffs overgrown with native plants, brush, and occasional wildflowers. Its paved path overlooked the bluffs and the Pacific Ocean. Walkers and joggers frequented the path all waking hours.

The ocean's scent would instantly invigorate me. Looking down over the bluffs and watching waves crashing in the dark made me feel as if I were visiting a resort.

Within days, I was able to sleep eight hours a day in shifts. The symptoms disappeared without sending me into depression. Minus the pain of exhaustion, I was able to make do with smoking one cigarette a week or less.

For the first time in my life, I had survived mild symptoms without them progressing into mania, without becoming severely depressed, and, miraculously, without medication. Once I got enough sleep, I do think that the hormones generated by nursing helped balance my biochemistry and helped keep more severe depression away.

The postpartum hormones had also caused hot flashes. Sudden, intense blasts of heat overtook my body and made me feel as if I had walked into a sauna. Hot flashes are a typical early postpartum symptom. What was strange about having hot flashes is that they made me realize I had experienced hot flashes at 19 during my first manic episode and during subsequent episodes. I had not known they were hot flashes. The waves of uncomfortable heat had seemed surreal like the rest of the symptoms.

During one of our daily strolls, I looked down at my not quite two-month-old son sleeping peacefully in his stroller and realized that, emotionally, I was not ready to hand over to daycare a tiny, helpless creature that couldn't even walk.

I ended up taking a year off from my job as a technical writer. As a first-time mother, the time off kept me from becoming overwhelmed. Spending time with my son doing the same mundane things over and over again until they became second nature made me more comfortable as a mother.

When my son was born, my relationship with my husband changed. There were things about Keith I could no longer ignore when I saw more of him and less of the world. We spent much more time together, and I became dependent on him both financially and for time to myself. I wanted my son to have the best of his father and began to realize I didn't know my husband that well. I didn't realize that I didn't know myself that well either.

I became distressed over some of my husband's choices. His behavior began to consume me. Once my son started eating baby food and I nursed less often, I also began struggling with mild depression. When I could no longer shake the mild depression with exercise, I decided to wean my seven-month-old son and resume taking lithium.

I found a therapist who, along with other friends, recommended a 12-step support group that taught me how to focus on myself and how to change my own thoughts and behavior instead of obsessing about others' unhealthy behavior. I also realized my job was not creatively or spiritually fulfilling, and I decided to change careers and become an elementary school teacher.

When my son turned one, I returned to work as a substitute school teacher and weighed about 145 pounds, a healthy weight for my toned 5' 7" frame.

I carefully arranged my leftover pasta, salad, chips, and oversized chocolate chocolate chip muffin in the order I would eat them. The fellow teacher sitting across from me in the teacher's cafeteria remarked in astonishment, "I have never seen anyone eat so much. How do you do it?"

I couldn't help but laugh, because he was only witnessing one of my five daily mega-meals. His blunt remark made me feel as if I were back in New York City. The comment was not mean-spirited. It was blurted out during the hurriedness of our brief lunch period.

In the course of nine months, I had transitioned from substitute teaching to long-term substitute teaching to a full-time position teaching elementary school. Getting my teaching credential while teaching full-time translated into working and going to school round the clock seven days a week for two and a half years. I did break to pick up my son and cook dinner every night.

By January 2001, my weight had crept up to over 190 pounds. In one year, I had gained 40 plus pounds.

Two afternoons a week I'd leave work at 3:30 instead of 5:30 and take my son to the park or the beach. By eight o'clock I was always back at the computer.

During the two years I attended my credential program, I stopped going to my support group, but, because I had had such a positive experience with that 12-step support group, I found my way once again to Overeater's Anonymous (OA). However, I was not able to change my eating habits even though I had made several short-lived attempts at abstinence (abstaining from compulsive overeating). Part of the reason those attempts failed was that I made too many drastic changes at once.

I had bought into our cultural view of eating disorders—you had a problem if you were full-blown anorexic, if you were 100 pounds or more overweight, or if you made yourself throw up on a regular basis. Ironically, I sought help for my compulsive eating addiction when it was less extreme than it had ever been. Letting myself be overweight had been huge progress for me because it meant I no longer alternated my bingeing with the starving that could trigger hypomania, although I did diet on and off.

What if? haunted me. *What if my job didn't work out? What if my marriage didn't work out?* Food temporarily quelled that nagging question that could haunt my thoughts. Food had become my tranquilizer, my sleeping pill, and my best friend.

CHAPTER 37

Greater-Than or Less-Than?

2001

While pursuing my teaching credential, I read about learning differences (a.k.a. processing challenges). Memories came flooding back of all the times I had hit a wall in certain subjects. I had never connected those incidents before.

1969

She had a limp. Curly hair and red lipstick sloppily applied. She scared me and every other second-grader in our class.

Math time was beginning. There was going to be a test soon. I didn't understand, yet again. I alternated staring at my paper, staring at the textbook, and staring at the board. I became self-conscious imagining that all my classmates could sense I had no idea what was going on.

While standing in line at the teacher's desk for help, I heard her helping the student in front of me. She said, "Think of the sign as the mouth of an alligator. The mouth opens to the larger number."

Suddenly I understood how to interpret greater-than and less-than signs—signs, which had been haunting me for two weeks. I slipped out of the line and was tempted to leap back to my desk, but settled for walking back instead.

"I said turn left," Keith has said to me too many times to count as I begin to turn in the wrong direction. I mix up left from right on a daily basis.

During dance class, I used landmarks, such as toward the piano and toward the door. I got by because once your body learns the moves and feels them in sync with the music, you do not need to think, instinct takes over.

Graphs are used throughout economics to show the relation-ship between variables, to take snapshots of economic data, and to explain complex ideas. It took me longer to read a graph than the average economics major but what derailed me was trying to draw the graphs. The tests for 400-level classes required you to draw graphs in order to explain the test questions. As soon as I would begin to draw, the graph would distort. I'd erase and flip it around back and forth and get hopelessly confused.

I had wanted to major in economics, but, instead, I made it my minor. By then, I was used to abandoning majors. If I had known about directional dyslexia, I might have been able to seek accommodations.

Directional dyslexia

Directional dyslexia is a term used to describe a variety of processing challenges that don't occur in the same combination for everyone with that diagnosis. It is a subset of dyslexia and involves fewer processing challenges than dyslexia.

For years, I chalked up my inability to retrieve words at times to exhaustion. I don't stutter, but when very tired, I kind of stammer. Sometimes, I can't spit out the right word. I can see an image in my mind, but I can't think of the word. *Could you give me the thing you measure with* (ruler)? *Where you go to get cash* (ATM).

My struggle gave me empathy for students who must figure out the accommodations they need to make in order to learn and all the adults who never figure out what they are up against, let alone how to accommodate their processing challenges.

Directional Dyslexia

Losing things
misplacing things
forgetting things

Writing on my wrist
so as not to forget.

Sometimes... still forgetting.
ANXIETY from forgetting...

Lists, lists, lists

Black accessory = lost accessory
Neon-green colored backpack
Scarlet red fake leather purse

Finally, learning faulty short-term memory
the culprit

Left, right, right, left, anxiety...
Disorientation
Hard to find parked car

Blue ink always when taking notes
Black ink jumbles.

CHAPTER 38

Sugar Sensitivity

Fall 2001

Becoming a parent was a revelation. I have never experienced more abundant joy than watching my child develop incrementally every day.

I don't think I will ever want anything more in this life than I wanted a second child. I desperately wanted a sibling for my son, and I sensed that, emotionally, it would be easier for me to parent two children instead of one. At 39, I had yet another miscarriage, and there wasn't much time left for me to conceive.

Summer 2002

In 1994, the real estate market had been at a low, and I had bought a foreclosed condo in Keith's building that we were able to rent out to a friend for well below market rate. Although I preferred the financial security of living below our means and owning a rental property, Keith refused to raise two children in a two-bedroom condominium with no yard. He also did not approve of the school in our semi-downtown school district, even though I had volunteered there and did approve of it.

In the summer of 2002, Keith and I sold both of our condos and bought a house.

My last miscarriage at 39 had brought me to the brink of despair. Although I had been healthy and free of psychotic episodes for years, I was frustrated, tremendously longing for a second child, and mourning all my miscarriages. Forty seemed like a death sentence because professionally I had not achieved my fiction writing goals.

Approaching the last hour of my biological clock, I sought salvation in the library and the Internet. I bought a book called *The Infertility Diet* by Fern Reiss that stressed nutrition as critical to promoting fertility. The book pointed out that, for some, extra weight could negatively impact fertility by throwing off estrogen levels and that rapidly gaining and losing weight could upset the delicate balance of reproductive hormones. It was painful to realize weight gain had not been the only price I had paid for my overindulgence.

Further research revealed that regularly consuming excessive amounts of sugar assaulted my cells subjecting them to chronic inflammation, which created a breeding ground for chronic disease.

Could I give up sugar for a chance at having another child?

Sugar. Tranquilizing. Intoxicating. My frenemy always screamed the same chant, "More, more, more." Chocolate, the most seductive of all, had become embedded in my molecules.

Icebox cake had once been my weekend go-to. Chocolate wafers layered with homemade whipped cream are placed in the refrigerator to emerge 12 hours later as a dessert that marries the bittersweet taste of chocolate with a luscious creaminess that keeps the sugar from overpowering the chocolate.

Even before my love affair with sugar ended, I had to stop making this inexpensive delicacy. Before I could share its 12 servings, I would eat the entire cake, one sloppy slice at a time, over the course of a few hours. I would tell myself each slice would be my last one.

And it was—for twenty minutes.

For years, whenever I had attended an Overeater's Anonymous (OA) meeting, I would hear, "Don't worry about giving up sugar. Your taste buds will change." I would nod my head and think, *Liar*.

Sugar had been my means of taking the edge off. When I overate, I numbed my feelings. Sugar was much safer than the prescription tranquilizers, anxiety erasers, which had once robbed me of my soul.

But that edge is what compels me to write. Finding my voice and sharing my voice hadn't been an issue, because I could not hear my own voice, well at least the voice of the creative soul within me. In part, I was so scared of mania that I somewhat censored myself when my thoughts wandered into story land.

"If you keep your food clean, things will come up," one of the OA speakers shared. Something got through.

The only way I could make peace with myself was to know that my eating habits were not keeping me from getting pregnant. If I could let go of binge eating, stabilize my weight, and eat healthy food, then I could accept not being able to give birth a second time. If I could not, *What if?* would forever haunt me.

I made one of those promises to the universe, that if I had a second child, I would never go back to my binge eating, yo-yo diets, and sugar orgies. I became abstinent from compulsive overeating on October 1, 2002.

I became abstinent to improve my chances of becoming pregnant and because I was sick of always being so vigilant and worrying something bad was going to happen. I was sick of myself and sought peace within myself.

At first, I defined my abstinence as not bingeing at night and following the food choices the book *Infertility Diet* by Fern Reiss recommended to optimize fertility.

Through working the steps, "things" came up. Sugar and white flour had kept me in a fog that kept me from feeling much of anything. Some research scientists purport that sugar is as addictive as cocaine and can be a gateway drug. Dr. DesMaisons' Radiant Recovery website is dedicated to treatment for sugar sensitivity and notes, "Sugar sensitive people feel pain more deeply and often use sugar to help quiet physical and emotional pain." The website describes sugar sensitivity as having three parts:

- Volatile blood sugar that overreacts to refined carbohydrates.

- Low levels of serotonin, the brain chemical that affects your mood and your ability to just say no.

- Low levels of beta-endorphin, the brain chemical that kills both physical and emotional pain.

The Friday night OA meeting I regularly attended was a speaker meeting. An opening speaker led the meeting and shared their experience, strength, and hope for about 15 minutes in addition to a guest speaker who shared for 30 minutes. I connected with many of the speakers' experiences.

I'm not religious, and God is a term I use by habit. My concept of God is that I can't fully understand the concept of God, but I can sense spiritual energy, life force, and light and connect with it.

I understand the concept of a higher power, which simply means I believe there is something in this universe more powerful than me. Nature is more powerful than me. The ocean. Wind. Wildflowers. Seagulls.

I can sense what I term light and dark, light being spiritual energy, and dark being the absence of spiritual energy. I can feel the love of a friend and the energy of the group at a 12-step meeting.

Sugar had been my savior at the age of five. It called to me. I had tried so many times to stop eating it. Try walking a block without encountering sugar. Coffee shops equal sugar. Well, okay, sugar and caffeine. Can you think of a more addictive equation?

There is sugar in the shoe store, hardware store, gas station, car dealership, and almost every establishment you enter.

Triggers. That delicate dance. I had to figure out what amount of sugar would not trigger the frenzy, the inability to stop ingesting desserts until I passed out or felt as I were about to explode. A teaspoon of sugar in my tea? Safe. Slightly sweet salad dressing? Careful. Oatmeal and strawberries? OK. But substituting dried fruit, such as those adorable dried apricots, was living dangerously.

It's always in the evening that I most crave something sweet to quell that feeling of anxiety about the many things I still need to get done that day. Sugar is not nearly as potent or tranquilizing as a Malibu Wave or Xanax, but it does work.

I developed alternate fixes to substitute for sugar. A bath so hot it causes me to shiver on immersion. Meditating by listening to a favorite song and absorbing it through movement. That one works well unless I wait until I am so exhausted that my brain freezes while trying to select a song. At that point, meditating is beyond me.

Giving up sugar and then white flour evolved from the gradual changes I made and working the steps. My despair motivated me. It took a few weeks for the intense cravings that howled, *More, more, more,* to diminish.

Within a few months, the craving, the overwhelming longing, subsided to mere desiring.

Eventually, my taste buds changed. Oatmeal, nuts, and strawberries or a slice of brown rice toast topped with almond butter, two grams worth of 85% Cacao dark chocolate fragments, apple slices, and cinnamon replaced homemade banana-and-more splits. I would smother the split banana with Ben and Jerry's New York Super Fudge Chunk ice cream, walnut pieces, and whipped cream.

I practiced stepping back and assessing what I was feeling. By allowing myself to experience the anxiety and discomfort sugar took away, deep-seated feelings of inadequacy and shame revealed themselves through journaling. Reflecting on my past relationships revealed a pattern of my behavior. I added the term emotionally unavailable man to my vocabulary.

I did not change overnight, but by dramatically changing the way I ate, I proved to myself I could change, which rejuvenated me and opened me up to possibility.

I did not change overnight, but by dramatically changing the way I ate, I proved to myself I could change, which rejuvenated me and opened me up to possibility.

I took my last final for my last teaching credential class in December 2002, and on Christmas Day, I learned I was pregnant.

To help release me from my obsession with my weight, I had begun weighing myself once a month instead of several times a day.

October 1, the scale read 186 pounds, and on January 1, it read 161 pounds.

CHAPTER 39

Feelings Return

Summer 2003

While walking toward the front door of our house, I noticed that the narrow front garden bordering our dusty peach stucco home had been disturbed.

My baby poppies had disappeared.

These weren't just any poppies. I had bought the seeds for the native California poppies at the Getty Museum months before and had patiently waited until the right time of year to plant them. I had provided them with nutrient-rich soil and tended to them. I had even said a prayer for them every day because a large tree shaded the front garden, and the shade threatened their survival. Somehow, the poppies had sprouted, and I had envisioned ribbons of orange, red, and yellow. I love poppies, because of the intensity of their color and their elegant simplicity.

Poppies look deliriously happy to me.

I found Keith watching TV and exclaimed, "What happened in the front yard? My poppies are gone."

"I thought they were weeds and pulled them," he replied.

I burst into tears and could not stop crying. I blubbered something to the effect, "How could you have? In all these months, haven't you heard a word I said about the poppies? How special they were to me.

"They can't be planted again for months, and they take months to sprout. You haven't done any yard work since we moved here."

Although I had learned I shouldn't play the martyr, that day I couldn't help myself. Between sobs, I stuttered, "I'm pregnant. I'm going to work, taking care of our son, dealing with all the contractors, and doing yard work when I'm so exhausted I can't even see straight, and you casually destroy my poppies.

"You never listen to me."

As soon as I began sobbing, Keith began walking away. I followed him around the house delivering my spiel as he furiously shut windows and angrily said, "The neighbors can hear you. You're embarrassing me."

The man was not listening to me at all, but I refused to let go. I wanted to make him understand how much he had hurt my feelings.

Pulling the poppies had been an accident, but that was not what upset me.

What upset me was that I had been gushing about those poppies for months, and he hadn't listened. He hadn't apologized. He hadn't offered to help me replace them. He had simply gotten angry and attacked me for caring so much about some almost-flowers.

That was my first real brush with abstinence. It was as if someone had turned on the volume and then turned up the volume.

Years later I can still remember the pain of that moment. I saw a part of Keith as he really was, at least, a part of him as he was in relationship to me at times, an angry, condescending man who dismissed my feelings, and it hurt so much.

Months later, in anger, he told me that day I had been psychotic—a curious choice of words to use with someone with my mental health history. Shocked, I had answered, "Why would you call me psychotic? Because I cried ugly, sobbed, for half an hour straight? Do you even know the definition of psychotic?"

His response had been to glare at me before saying, "You know you hit me that day."

"Hit you! I don't remember that. All I remember is you shaking me while I was in the bathroom. You were trying to get me to stop crying, and I struggled to get your arms off of me. Is that what you call hitting?"

He had shrugged in disgust and walked away.

I don't cry often, but that day my entire body had shuddered and sobs had emerged from deep within.

I'm not a name caller. My experience with my father made me loathe to call anyone names. In anger, Keith called me a variety of derogatory names. Often, I laughed off the put-downs and responded with, "It's time to play "Clock the Criticisms" again. A new record. Five put-downs in 30 seconds."

Sometimes, I simply ignored his demands for a perfectly clean house, perfectly behaved kids, perfect meals, and a perfect paycheck.

Looking back, that day I saw that Keith was a stranger to me in many ways, but I did not want to accept that. I knew right then and there I wanted out unless Keith changed. And I'd been letting go of trying to force him to change for four years. So, I prayed. I still held out hope that if I changed enough, became more accepting, more enlightened, and healthier, Keith would become less angry.

That day I felt betrayed. Working through that feeling without overeating was uncomfortable, and, to an extent, I put aside my feelings. I accepted that Keith was not capable of understanding the depth of my emotion and that part of me judged myself more harshly than even he did.

Once I stopped overeating and doing step work, I'd have flashbacks of past incidents with Keith that made me realize that all along Keith had been showing me who he was beneath his mask, and I had chosen not to see the parts of him I didn't want to see. Subconsciously, the masochist in me, the pain junkie, had not been fazed by his rage.

One flashback played in my head as if it had happened yesterday. Before we were married, Keith, one of his friends, and I attended a U2 concert at Anaheim Stadium. It was one of those concerts that achieved theater. The staging, the stage presence and intensity of the musicians, the lighting, and above all the music infused me with positive energy, and I walked out of the concert feeling very much alive.

That is until we got to the parking lot. Keith and his friend fell into the car and promptly passed out.

I had to drive Keith and his friend 20 miles home in intense fog with almost no visibility.

After dropping them off, I couldn't find a parking spot. I had given up my parking spot in my building to his visiting friend.

By 1 a.m., I had been driving around my neighborhood for over an hour. I was getting spooked as I lived three blocks from an urban park that housed meth addicts after midnight. I drove to Keith's condo, rang his buzzer until I woke him up, and asked him to help me. He became enraged that I had woken him up and begrudgingly moved his friend's car.

At the time I was livid and even slapped his face once, which upset me more than him because it was so against my code of conduct given my childhood experience. The next day I forgave him. I should have called him on his chosen behavior and whether he was comfortable living like that every weekend. He had traveled into another dimension and had jettisoned any regard for my welfare and safety. What's on me, I realized from step work, is that I enabled this behavior by accepting it.

Keith had many positive qualities that had attracted me too, and he showed me love as well as rage. However, the rage rattled me and triggered feelings of fear and helplessness from childhood.

Many memories returned in abstinence from compulsive eating. Releasing addiction can be summed up in six words…

Learning how to *feel it now.*

The behavior or the substance, the addiction, served as my mechanism toward attempting to *feel it never.*

Excessive amounts of food had numbed the aching emptiness from within. While manic and single, impulsivity ruled me, and I used drugs and sex with strangers to numb my pain.

Mania is akin to undergoing a personality transplant. I remember finding some of my male classmates attractive and witty as far back as junior high school. I still find certain men attractive, but I have zero desire to pursue one-night stands. It's not restraint or age, I have always been that way when not under the influence of drugs or mania. It was not at all challenging to be faithful to my husband for 17 years.

If I keep myself away from individuals who habitually use drugs and practice the principles of my program, keeping clean is not a struggle either. However, sugar and bread are still a bit of a daily challenge.

Why doesn't conventional psychiatry address the influence of addiction? Treat the mind, body, and spirit and not only the mind? In Canada, mental health and addiction are now treated together.

There are many complementary remedies to balance brain chemistry, such as exercise, meditation, massage, and nutrition. Choosing friends, careers, and a lifestyle that supports my health has been critical as has getting to know my body's signals.

Subtle mood changes are my body's way of telling me it's craving more sleep and less stimulation. If I start raising my voice, I now know I need to take a walk, to rest, or to be around less stimulation even if that means not running errands, cleaning the house, or honoring social obligations. This insight has enabled me to stay on an amount of medication I can tolerate without being overwhelmed by the unpleasant side effects that kept me from taking the medication regularly.

The spiritual component of healing is difficult to describe, but it has helped me change the way I think, the hardest thing I have ever had to do. Negative thinking is the worst culprit. The more I focus on gratitude and live in the moment, the more I enjoy life.

My repetitive negative thoughts have morphed over the years. As I write this, I realize that it has been 11 years since persistent depression kept me trapped in negative thoughts that looped throughout the day for days. But there are times, such as after Daylight Saving Time, when the negative thoughts creep back. By now, I have an arsenal of tools to combat incipient depression, including exercise. Mainly, I worry about finances. What if I lost my job in the midst of another recession? What if I can't help my kids get through college?

Recovery taught me how to accept the inner turmoil and how to identify my part in creating it so I could learn how to identify and accept what was within my control and not create as much turmoil. Working the steps and the recovery process also taught me that sometimes turmoil is a sign I am headed in the wrong direction.

And then there's my sensitive biochemistry. The slightest uncertainty, generally about whether my job will last, and I develop a knot in my chest and a feeling of dread—mild depression. The irony is that I struggle with this more since abstinence. I used to eat at night to the point of passing out, which resulted in my not feeling much of anything.

Learning about the sensory sensitivity processing trait, a.k.a. highly sensitive, has helped me understand my empathy, my sensitivity to sound, and my keen observations. It also sparked the memory of what my ninth grade English teacher wrote in my yearbook, "Those with sensitive insight will leave a marked impression on this world."

Seeking external substances or compulsive behaviors to quell internal turmoil is one way to define addiction.

Recovery taught me how to let go, surrender, and act "as if." Act as if everything will work out. Carry on even though I feel like crap. Accept that I cannot possibly imagine every possible permutation of circumstances that would enable things to work out or how exactly they will work out. Am I batting a thousand on this process? *No.* Or, if I put on my optimist hat, I would answer, *Not yet.*

CHAPTER 40

Colic

2003

Once a week during my pregnancy with my second child, I found myself in a room down the hall from my doctor's office hooked up to a machine that was able to monitor whether my body was experiencing minor contractions. It caught them twice. Each time minor medical intervention and a bout of bed rest got the pregnancy back on track.

Close to my due date, my water broke, and my contractions speeded up so quickly that we were on our way to the hospital within an hour. We arrived at the hospital around 10 p.m., and I was certain my daughter would not arrive until the next day.

Even though my contractions indicated it was time for me to deliver my infant, my cervix was not dilated nearly enough. The same thing had happened to me with my son, and it had taken one and a half days, anesthesia, and, finally, induced labor to achieve dilation.

I couldn't imagine going through that ordeal again, and I started silently praying to my mother and begging her to help me.

Forty minutes later, Laura came into this world so quickly that she was born bright pink and well before midnight.

It felt as if the heavens had opened and dropped her into my outstretched 41-year-old arms.

The following day, presenting my curious four-year-old son with a sister filled me with joy that warmed my entire body. I will never want anything in life more than I wanted my first child and then my second child.

My daughter had colic, and it was a challenge to get enough sleep. Unlike my experience with my firstborn, my body instantly produced milk, and nursing her was easy.

When my daughter was not quite a month old, I went through a jug of Red Vines in three days and realized how vulnerable I still was to the allure of sugar. I began planning my meals again and reaffirmed my commitment to keeping sugar out of my food plan.

But the thing about sugar is that it worked. It reduced my anxiety. Without it, or any other substance, my anxiety became very uncomfortable. How was I going to go back to teaching elementary school and nurse my infant in mere weeks? It was a bad plan.

The hormones from the pregnancy and the joy of being pregnant had made me feel calm and confident. I had forgotten how depression and anxiety felt and had overlooked the impossible logistics of pumping milk while teaching elementary school.

I struggled with postpartum depression and returned to therapy for the first time in years. The sessions helped me reframe my catastrophic thinking.

I was learning to focus on the positive aspects of my relationship with my husband and life in general. For emotional support, I had friends and an infinite amount of support from my two programs, and I was learning how to provide emotional support to myself.

I did not feel as if I received much emotional support from Keith, but he pitched in and helped with our children on the occasions I asked him. I don't want to paint the wrong picture of Keith. He has probably missed one day of work in the last 20 years.

However, we are on different wavelengths. If I had worked through the 12 steps before we met, we never would have gotten married.

Other than the few sessions I had with a therapist after my son was born, I hadn't been in therapy since saying good-bye to Sarah in 1991. When I stopped overeating, I became an open wound, and I realized sugar and white flour had served as my tranquilizer.

When my daughter was 10 weeks old, I began planning for my return to work after Christmas vacation. I intended to pump milk, store it, and nurse on my classroom breaks. This was an absurd plan as was my plan to return to work so quickly. Friends of mine begged me to take the medical leave of absence my psychiatrist was offering me that would allow me to stay home until the following school year began, but I didn't want my students to spend their entire year with substitute teachers or create a hassle for the school.

Over the phone, I discussed taking a medical leave of absence with a union representative who said, "If you take a medical leave of absence related to bipolar disorder, you will never get your job back." I didn't realize until years later that he had been absolutely wrong as the details of my medical leave of absence would have been confidential due to HIPAA (Health Insurance Portability and Accountability Act).

After my sugar frenzy, the postpartum depression had only lasted about two weeks but had yielded me Rita, a therapist with whom I felt comfortable. The Monday of the week of Thanksgiving, I started pumping extra breast milk in preparation for my return to work.

I slid into severe depression within three days, more quickly than I ever had in my life.

Thanksgiving morning, I was having visions of Keith as a widower, depressed and struggling to take care of two children on his own.

You're worthless. You don't deserve to live, and you'll never be able to function again. If you wean your daughter abruptly, she'll be psychologically scarred for life, was the chorus that raced through my thoughts.

I felt light-headed and overwhelmed. I called a friend, a mother of three, and confessed that I felt like a failure.

She told me that she saw a loving, capable mother and to please forget about feeling guilty about weaning my daughter, she wouldn't be the first baby whose mother had a medical emergency and couldn't nurse her. She also told me not to feel ashamed about needing to call my doctor on Thanksgiving Day.

I called my doctor.

I had weaned my son during a two-week period, but I weaned my daughter during the course of Thanksgiving Day so I could immediately resume lithium. She would not take a bottle from me for a day and a half. Keith and our friends gave her bottles, and she ate well.

Laura did let me hold her, but she scowled at me at first.

Within hours of taking lithium, my thoughts slowed down a bit. Within 10 days of resuming lithium, I felt like myself.

I never stopped using my other tools to avoid depression. These other tools, such as exercise, prayer, meditation, keeping my blood sugar on an even keel, and writing a gratitude list daily enabled me to maintain on a dose of lithium I can tolerate without traveling to Zombieville and losing all cognitive function except the ability to sort laundry all day.

These tools also enabled me to return to full functioning once the lithium kicked in rather than struggle for weeks or months with mild or moderate depression.

Within one month back at work, I knew I would resign my teaching position effective when the school year ended. I had gotten confident after the first child, but colic was an entirely higher level of challenge as was returning to teaching after four months instead of 12 months.

The decision to resign brought me much anguish, because I loved teaching and had worked hard to get my credential. I had been reassigned from third grade to fifth grade. My class size went from 20 to 30 students, and I was in over my head with 50% more inner-city students who were approaching puberty. Teaching involved long hours. I could do most of the grading and lesson planning from my home, but my infant daughter needed constant attention and still woke up in the middle of the night because of her colic.

Because of the incessant crying, some nights I would get four hours of sleep. My reaction time was so impaired, I was terrified of running my car off the road.

Although I was only experiencing mild symptoms of depression intermittently, I was sleep-deprived and felt exhausted, frazzled, forgetful, and a beat behind most of the time. Being tired made me less efficient, and the 50 odd hours a week I worked were simply not enough to feel as organized and confident as I needed to feel to be an effective teacher.

My class was mostly boys, and most of them played me for a sucker. Newer teachers always get some of the most challenging students. I had had good luck with reaching defiant girls, but not as much reaching the mischievous boys.

During the lessons such as math, art, writing, and science in which I could include hands-on activities and lecture the least amount possible—quick lesson, model the lesson, monitor the students as they executed the lesson—the classroom generally hummed. The reading program did not hum.

CHAPTER 41

Step Work

August 2004

A little voice inside me prompted me to approach an old-timer who was available to sponsor. Rene, an AA and OA veteran, had a reputation for being tough. I almost talked myself out of approaching her, because she followed a much more stringent food plan than I did, which included meat, vegetables, and not much else.

"What do you need help with?"

"The steps."

Rene never asked me about my food plan. Shortly thereafter, I gave up white flour. Although the cravings were not as bad as those from sugar, eating breadsticks, pizza, pasta, and the like made me hungry again shortly thereafter.

While working the steps, I began coming to terms with why I had such intense shame about my past sexual behavior. A memory came up.

At the end of the summer between 9th and 10th grade, I was 14 and had returned home in disgrace from my summer job as a mother's helper. The summer had gone well, except that I had puzzled the first-time 40ish mother of a two-and-a-half-year-old. I can still picture the astonished look on her face when she said, "The cooking, the sewing, the decorating. How do you do all of this on your day off? It is exhausting to watch you."

What had gotten me in trouble at summer's end was that I had stayed out late at a party, and a man in his forties who had been chaperoning his friend's son had given me and two other teens a ride home.

The man had not flirted with me, let alone made a pass at me, but somehow my father had found out about the ride home. Once I returned home, my father had hauled me to the police station. While I sat there, he had a LONG conversation with the police officer about whether he could press charges and the grounds for pressing charges for sexual molestation and statutory rape.

The message had come through loud and clear—lose my virginity or anything close before my 18th birthday, and my father would press charges against the boy or man whether the charges would stick or not.

My father punished me for staying out late by not allowing me to be on the gymnastics team during 10th grade.

I had learned gymnastics from watching it on television. Although I had grown up in apartments, I practiced handstands against my closet door and seized every chance I got to practice on any lawn I came across. On my own, I had mastered cartwheels, handstand forward rolls, front walkovers, and front handsprings.

My freshman year, I did not compete, but the gymnastics coach had patiently worked with me. I had been getting used to the low balance beam and was learning back walkovers by leaning backward into a bridge and then pushing my feet off against a wall.

Not being allowed to return to the gymnastics team devastated me.

The memory of the police station made me squirm but remembering the earlier part of that day made me laugh. My father had picked me up at Penn Station in Manhattan. During the walk to Grand Central Station through midtown Manhattan, his anger had propelled him into a temper tantrum. Halfway to our destination, he had abruptly halted, turned toward me, and said, "Give me your check."

I obediently opened my backpack and silently handed over my summer earnings check over. He put down my duffel bag that he had been carrying and then proceeded to grab my backpack from me and rummage through it until he found my curling iron. He extricated it from my tangle of hastily packed shorts, T-shirts, and toiletries. He held it out in front of him as if he were about to conduct a symphony with it.

Amidst many passersby on a midtown sidewalk and with great flair, my father had lifted up the slender wand of metal and plastic, held it across his thigh, and snapped it in two. Then, with a flourish, he threw the two pieces into a trashcan.

I was so embarrassed, I became unembarrassed.

It was akin to getting desensitized. By 14, I was used to his outbursts. The absurdity of his stunt on a crowded midtown street stunned me, but then it amused me. I could picture how unreal and theatrical it must have looked to anyone passing by. I didn't dare laugh.

Being in public on a midtown street had saved me from getting kicked, slapped, or thrown against a wall. I prayed that his rage had been spent for the day and that he would return to simply leaving me on my own much of the time.

The next day, I rescued the letter from my father's trashcan that had accompanied me home. The mom had said many complimentary things about me, including, "Sasha seems much older than 14, I forget that she is 14."

The first time I remember my father leaving me alone was on a Saturday night. I was nine years old. We were living in a faculty apartment complex in a small college town in Wisconsin. I felt safe there and was excited to be on my own all night.

Often, my father left me in the hands of others, and they were always good people. In junior high, we lived in Astoria, Queens, a working-class neighborhood a 20-minute subway ride from midtown Manhattan. There were three units in our building. Our apartment occupied the top story, the third story. Our landlords had one child, a daughter my age. Their apartment occupied the second story, and a foyer and smaller apartment took up the ground floor. The building also included a finished basement, which our landlords mainly used for entertaining guests. They heard my fathers' rages, and their response had been to open their home to me. I was often there after school and spent many weekends with them in their weekend home in Rocky Point, New York.

The summer after seventh grade, my father sent me to France to visit with my sixth-grade au pair, Michelle, and her family. The goal was to perfect my limited French. Michelle's three sisters competed for who would get to spend time with me. One sister taught me how to make salad dressing from scratch.

Another sister taught me how to flirt. She said, "When you see a cute young man, you approach him and ask him for the time. But you don't say it like that. Do something like pointing to your wrist and say, 'That which you have on your wrist. Which numbers are being pointed to?'"

I learned how much fun being silly could be.

Michelle also imported Katharine, her 11-year-old cousin, to hang out with me. Katharine was full of mischief despite her quiet demeanor. During a tour of a museum, she faked a stomach virus. By the time her squirming morphed into groans and fake heaves, she had enlisted me to join her.

To my shock, the middle-aged museum-goers turned around and clapped. They burst into laughter and encouraged us to continue.

That could never have happened in the United States. French culture can be described in two words. Pourquoi pas? Why not?

CHAPTER 42

Sylvia

March 2005

I quit drinking because I noticed that most of the people who achieved long-term abstinence from compulsive overeating did not drink. Alcohol had never been my drug of choice. I had occasionally abused it when nothing else had been around, but that had not been for 12 years. However, lithium intensified the effect of alcohol by at least double. I averaged a couple of drinks a couple of times a week, which made me loose. And I had been hanging on to those couple of days a week.

I never realized what alcohol did for me until I gave it up. Anxiety flooded me.

Pink polka dots appeared on my face. They got bigger and bigger until I finally sought medical advice. What I heard was, "Could cause permanent scarring," and, "If it is the lithium, and you stop taking lithium, the rash won't disappear right away. The allergy has taken on a life of its own."

Lithium can cause skin rashes, and I decided to switch medications. My psychiatrist, Dr. Kandy, recommended Abilify. Psychiatric medications vary in the amount of time in which they can take effect. Sometimes it can take a few weeks. I have heard of patients responding wonderfully to Abilify, but it made me retch and then dry heave all night long. One night, on the way to the bathroom I stumbled and fell facedown, bruising my forehead. After one week of barely sleeping, I gave up and asked Dr. Kandy if there was a slow-release version of Tegretol. There was, and I switched to it.

Without mentioning it to Dr. Kandy, to compensate for not having slept much the week I was on Abilify, I also started taking the Dalmane I had never thrown out from my Thanksgiving postpartum episode. I had only needed several days' worth of the 30-day prescription to get back on track sleep-wise when my daughter had been an infant.

Within a couple of days, I needed the Dalmane during the day to relax and to nap—I craved it constantly. I craved how Dalmane fixed everything. It provided an absolute mental vacation.

I realized I was having symptoms again because I now had trouble sleeping without Dalmane. I felt speeded up, I was losing weight without trying, and I could not easily concentrate. Keith tells me that during this period I woke him up in the middle of the night every night to have sex. At first, I did not see the Dalmane as contributing to my hypomania.

Probably because I no longer overate, drank, or smoked, once I started taking Dalmane, I craved tranquilizers and weed badly. I hadn't craved drugs so strongly in 12 years and was scared.

I found my way to an NA meeting on the beach adjacent to Bluff Park. Comforted by the beauty of the jagged rocks that made up the bluff and the accents of color the native plants provided, I found the courage to approach a street-smart woman close to my age, Sylvia, who agreed to sponsor me. I didn't consider Dalmane a drug. I needed it to sleep. I needed to sleep to prevent mania. I was worried about smoking weed.

Not every person with bipolar disorder who uses sleeping pills is a drug addict. However, anyone coping with bipolar disorder needs regular sleep to avert mania, depression, or both.

After teaching, I had returned to work as a contract technical writer. It was less demanding than teaching, and I found it easier to balance motherhood with technical writing.

Sylvia and I met early Sunday mornings and she began taking me page by page through the Big Book. I finally got the three-fold nature of addiction. I had always understood the physical part and somewhat the mental and spiritual parts, but never the power of the subconscious.

If I had trouble sleeping, why the Hell was I cleaning the house at 3 a.m. when I woke up? Why was I heading to the computer and writing then? I realized that the addict within wanted to drive me to exhaustion, to the brink of mania, so that sleeping pills were justified.

In a moment of clarity, I realized Dalmane had triggered the restlessness, the hypomania I had been fighting off for a couple of weeks, and my craving for more tranquilizers. I realized that eventually, I would be craving street drugs too, and I was doomed if I didn't give up the Dalmane.

Oct. 23, 2005, was my first day without Dalmane. I was shaky for a week, but I used the same breathing and relaxation routine I had used after my son was born, and I was able to sleep through the night fairly quickly.

I had two kids. I had averted mania for 12 years and succumbed only once in 17 years. The fighter in me took over. The Dalmane had caused the only hypomanic episode I had experienced since 1993 other than my brief postpartum brushes with hypomania.

I got that using drugs, even once, threatened my mental health. Just as my system had little tolerance for most psychiatric drugs, it had even less tolerance for street drugs.

Even more than before, I designed my life to enhance regular sleep. I am relieved that on the rare occasions when necessary, once or twice a year, a low dose of the antihistamine Benadryl can help me sleep. Benadryl at bedtime has been easing my seasonal hay fever symptoms since childhood without any side effects except drowsiness. However, if I need Benadryl simply to help me sleep, I take it as a red flag that it's time to lighten my schedule a bit.

Willingness to be open to whatever change is needed makes room for growth, but the willingness has to be constantly reinforced.

Willingness to be open to whatever change is needed makes room for growth, but the willingness has to be constantly reinforced.

Sylvia begged me to read the book *The Power of Now*. When I read, "You are not your mind," a wave of relief flooded through me that has never quite left. I got how, to a great extent, I create my life and how I create drama at times. Between the countless fourth-step inventories of my feelings and behavior I had done with Rene, working with Sylvia, and reading *The Power of Now*, I slowly started becoming comfortable in my own skin.

The Power of Now gave me new tools. These tools don't work magic for me, but they do help:

- There is a difference between my ego and my soul.

- In a sense, problems are an illusion.

- Completely engaging in the moment eradicates anxiety.

- Being in your body, instead of only in your head, helps connect you to your soul.

I started attending a women's meeting of Cocaine Anonymous called "Removing the Mask." Cocaine had not been my thing, but it was a rare women's meeting, and at a convenient time and location.

Some of the women who attended had left behind years of crack addiction and had completely rebuilt their lives. Their strength and faith permeated the room.

Newly sober I confessed, "I slept with 50 men, and I'm so ashamed."

"I think I slept with those same 50 men." Laughter.

The words had come from a woman with stringy long hair and granny glasses who was missing a tooth. From the twinkle in her eyes, I could see her as she had once been. Drug addiction had claimed her looks but no longer claimed her sense of humor.

CHAPTER 43

On Stage

2006

At 17, I had toyed with the idea of becoming a professional dancer. At 18, I slept through my college dance concert never again to appear on stage as a dancer.

Three and a half years after abstaining from compulsive overeating, I attended the March 2006 Erma Bombeck Writer's Workshop in Dayton, Ohio. In preparation for the conference, I joined their online humor writing group. I had been writing screenplays for seven years, including comedies. But with two children, I realized Hollywood was too hard to navigate, and I wanted to write and syndicate a humor column. *The World's Laziest Mommy* was a self-deprecating column poking fun at all my shortcuts, such as having my son and his friend play "General Contractor" to trick them into completing chores. After writing a half-dozen sample columns, I realized the theme was better suited to fiction and that in order to churn out an original column every week that held my interest, I would have to also make it informative.

Scrimping to Splurge, another potential column, would discuss not so drastic ways to save money and time, how to have fun being frugal, and how to make time to pursue passions. Unfortunately, my timing was not the best. Newspapers were declining.

"There are a couple more slots open for the closing night comedy show. Is anyone brave enough? You only have to perform seven minutes," was posted in the online forum six weeks before the conference.

I couldn't resist the challenge, even though I had not set foot on a stage for over two decades and had never before performed stand-up, let alone in front of close to 100 people.

Canadian author and entertainer Gordon Kirkland organized the show and advised me to rehearse a lot. I did.

My two-year-old daughter and my seven-year-old son were my practice audience. It was easy to make them laugh back then.

Buy the cheapest house in the best neighborhood. Great advice.

Now my kids think they're underprivileged because we don't weekend in Maui.

"Mommy, why don't we have a housekeeper?"

"We do. It's you. Here's your broom. Get going."

My son goes on a playdate with Jake. They take him to Disneyland.

Jake comes to our house, and I take them to the living room.

But I make them stand in line and pay me five bucks each.

At the conference's comedy show, I was the only comic who performed some jokes about writing, and the audience of writers howled with laughter.

Writing beats some of my former addictions.

Now, if I could only become addicted to marketing… I might actually sell something.

That night and the next morning, some of the attendees approached me to compliment my performance, and one attendee said, "I love your Spacey L.A. Mom act." I thanked her and thought to myself, *I'm lucky someone else figured out my act because I never would be able to.*

I discovered an entirely new way to experience excitement without taking drugs or having an affair with an elusive man. Stand-up comedy also helped me cope with my frustration about not getting regularly published as a fiction writer.

"Keith called me a whore," I lamented to Rene.

"Why does that bother you?" she responded. I thought to myself, *What is it with this woman? Is she crazy? Why wouldn't that bother me?* I can't remember what I answered.

"If some part of you didn't believe that was true, it wouldn't bother you this much. I'm not saying that you should like him calling you a whore, but that you have to recognize your feelings and accept them," Rene added.

Her response got me thinking.

Writing countless inventories rewired my thought patterns. I learned to write about: what happened, how what happened made me feel, what I feared, and what I could do to change. Those inventories made me aware of the daily choices I make to which I had never given much thought. They also made me step back and try to be objective instead of letting events eat away at me and instead of becoming more and more upset.

For example, I hated when one of my family members screamed at me or seethed at me, but by answering them back, I had taught them it was OK to scream at me.

Instead of screaming back, storming off, or twisting myself into a pretzel to avoid topics that would make them scream, I learned that I could calmly respond, "I can't talk to you when you scream at me." I also learned the effect their anger had on me. I could feel it in my body, particularly in my chest. Having kept myself numb with food had kept me from experiencing their disapproval and anger.

Anger is like fire, it needs to be fed. By learning how not to react, their anger often dwindled. And humor can be effective in disarming an angry person.

Years later, I fully understand what Rene meant. If all it takes for me to turn to dust is for someone to say, "You're a slut," or "You're crazy," then I'm easily manipulated. If I'm living my life just to prove wrong anyone who might say that, then that's wasted energy.

"Don't take anything personally," is the third agreement in Don Miguel Ruiz's best-seller *The Four Agreements: A Toltec Wisdom Book*.

I developed a different set of eyes through each addiction I released. While in remission from bipolar depression, my addictions were not dramatic, but they kept me from experiencing much joy. They kept me from getting to know my true purpose, and they kept me stagnant.

For me, recovery was akin to waking up and becoming one person.

So many memories returned in abstinence and sobriety that I was able to remember what once I had blocked out or buried. Those memories often made me gulp for air and cause tightness in my upper chest near my heart.

Releasing the buried pain made room for growth.

Depression distorted my thinking, but in a weird way, it made it clearer. Depression stripped me of the focus on daily tasks, the busyness, that allowed me to stay in denial. Shoving down feelings and willing everything to be OK had become a way of life to me. During the depression, I often had insights into other individuals' dark sides, but I had neither the faith that I could make it on my own without them nor the energy to make necessary changes.

During marriage counseling, I learned that I tend to see people for who they could become, not for who they are. I am aware now that I will always have the potential to "fix" friends, lovers, and relatives.

Although I went into mourning after resigning from my teaching position, my only paid job that used all of my innate talents, Keith was angry for years over my walking away from a secure, relatively well-paying job that synced better with the children's schedules. He had never understood that I had been past the brink of exhaustion when I resigned, that my mental health had been at stake, and most importantly, at the time, I did not have the stamina to teach fifth grade, the grade to which I had been reassigned, and would have been shortchanging my students.

Rene had said to me once, "He has the right to be an asshole." I can't remember what we were discussing. She meant it's not up to me to decide what's best for anyone else but myself. I can have an opinion, but it's up to that individual and the energy of the cosmos to help that individual choose their own destiny.

Whenever an acquaintance's behavior mystifies me or disappoints me, I can hear

People are just being who they are.

209

Rene's voice in my head saying to me, "People are just being who they are." Then I silently thank her. She said that to me on several occasions, but I can't remember the situations that prompted that particular remark of hers.

"People are just being who they are," is another way of saying, "Don't take it personally." It works better for me because it takes the focus off of me and reminds me that some people are coming from a different place and may have different values or standards of behavior.

When I lamented to Rene about family members not supporting my decisions, she replied, "You don't need anyone's approval, but your own." During our step work, I learned that I went to great lengths to please friends and relatives because I sought their approval.

The problem was that my neediness for approval obscured my getting to know myself, my needs, and my wants. I'm not talking about compassion or empathy—those are gifts. I'm talking about subconsciously manipulating other people's feelings. What other people thought of me had become more important to me than what I thought of myself, because it had become too painful to face my fears.

CHAPTER 44

Transitions

I felt shaky driving with my new medication. The previous version of this particular medication had always made me very light-headed, but almost the entire time I had taken that version of the medication, I had lived in New York City and rarely had to drive.

At Bellevue, I had shared a room with a young woman my age, Maria, and we had become close friends. Since Bellevue, she had been in and out of hospitals and had seen many prominent psychiatrists in New York City. She had raved about a different anticonvulsant, and I had switched to it with my new doctor. The therapeutic dose of it knocked me out cold, made me very sleepy, and I had been taking a "baby dose" of it.

My new doctor worked part-time at the practice I visited. At one point, I had to wait over two weeks to visit her. At the time, I met with my therapist about once a month. Before I could utter the word depression during my visit, my therapist read my mind and said, "Would you feel more comfortable with your old doctor?" I swallowed my pride and said, "Yes."

I was able to see Dr. Kandy within a few days and resumed lithium about three weeks from the onset of depression. My rash had been gone for months. Within two weeks of resuming lithium, the depression lifted. For those three weeks, I had been using every tool I had ever adopted to keep functioning and remain cheerful around my children, but that episode made me respect bipolar disorder even more. However, I believe that using tools, such as keeping a gratitude journal and exercise at least kept me functioning during the depression.

The security I feel from having a psychiatrist I trust readily available is immense. I don't need to see my psychiatrist often, every three to four months generally, but if my health is threatened, immediately consulting with a medical professional can be the difference between a blip and a breakdown.

November 2006

My logic was that I had no control over Keith, and, as a working mom, somewhat limited control over my income, so I was going to let go and focus on the parts of my life that brought me joy—my children, my writing, my job, stand-up comedy, volunteering, and my friends.

I gave up trying to find a position that paid a salary that matched my education, skills, and experience. Many technical writing jobs are located in Irvine, only 24 miles from Long Beach. But you can't get on the road after 6:00 a.m. in the morning or after 3 p.m. in the afternoon unless you like driving seven miles an hour and a 90-minute or more each way commute. Commuting stress, and the stress of feeling that I was neglecting my children, given their ages at the time, were deadly to me, yet I interviewed for these jobs.

I took a different approach and focused on finding a job within a ten-mile radius from home, and I found a job within one month. It paid 20 percent less than the jobs I had been interviewing for, but I took comfort in knowing that plenty of other working moms have traded away more income for less commute and more time with their children.

After five years of having 12-step programs as my priority, I stepped back, but not away. I only had a few hours to myself a week and needed a creative outlet. Rene, Sylvia, and the other sponsors I have had gave me an awareness of my thoughts, feelings, and behaviors that I continue to learn from and apply when I remember to step back from incidents so I can assess my part and evaluate what I need to accept or what I need to change.

Sometimes, what seems like a disappointment is a blessing in disguise. For example, landing in Bellevue seemed to be the absolute worst day of my life, but it turned out to be the best thing that ever happened to me in terms of finally getting comprehensive, effective mental health treatment.

April 2008

When the pink polka dots on my face returned, I made an appointment with my general practitioner.

By the time my appointment arrived, the splotches had faded. I sat on an examining table as the doctor bent closer and moved his head around as he scanned my face. Then he stood up and didn't say anything. I could tell he was thinking.

"They were worse last week," I said. Because he was still silent, I kept talking, "Also, I was fighting off a cold."

The doctor scrunched his mouth slightly and said, "I think you have rosacea. Rosacea is affected by your immune system."

Relief washed over me. If it was rosacea, then it wasn't the lithium, and I wouldn't have to give up the lithium again.

Two days later, I remembered that I used to occasionally get nervous rashes as a teenager that were caused by stress or scented soap.

August 2008

Relationships involve compromise, but they shouldn't involve checking your soul in a closet every time you are together.

My wedding day was one of the happiest days of my life. If I had known myself better, I never would have married Keith. However, he believed in me when I didn't believe in myself.

His predictability, stability, and affection were good for me. My spontaneity, warmth, and humor were good for him.

When one person changes in a relationship, the relationship is bound to change. Ultimately, I filed for divorce from my husband, because his lifestyle became incompatible with mine. Our differences threatened my mental health and my clean time.

I've come to accept that along with being energetic and enthusiastic when well-rested, I'm also excitable and defensive when stressed. When I meditate regularly, I find myself able to relax and not react so quickly.

Although I attended my first 12-step meeting, NA, at 23, I didn't work my first 12-step program until I was 37 years old. Through working the steps, my spiritual energy changed significantly. In order to not use food, drugs, sex, compulsive relationships, anything external to escape the loneliness, emptiness, fear, or whatever discomfort I'm experiencing, I had to connect with my spirit—who I truly am. Not who I think I should be.

When I'm having an anxious day, I sometimes use this affirmation, "I am safe. I am healthy. God is love. I feel love." And then I feel the wind, notice the beauty of a plant, or feel the warmth of my child's smile, and I feel comfort. I feel alive. Sometimes it works long enough to tide me over until I get immersed in work or housework.

When I'm having a frustrating day, and I need a laugh, I say to myself, *If the ghost of Cary Grant were to stroll into my life today, how much would my life really change? Would he write my short stories for me? Would he convince editors to publish my articles? Would he mother my children? Would he make me happy?*

No one can make me happy, but me. But I wouldn't mind having dinner with a debonair ghost.

CHAPTER 45

Will Effective Treatment for Addiction Ever Become the Norm?

(DrivenToTellStories.com blog, October 2016)

Addiction is complex, yet simple. Addiction enables you to avoid uncomfortable feelings by escaping your reality. Addiction lives in the subconscious and masks your soul. It is fueled by denial.

The Atlantic's April 2015 article, "The Irrationality of AA" by Gabrielle Glaser reveals seldom talked about treatment options for addiction, but its title is curious.

Alcoholics Anonymous (AA) and all the 12-step programs are spiritual programs. Spirituality, faith, is the opposite of rationality. Faith is based on believing in that which cannot be proven or seen, whereas rationality is based on facts, the tangible.

The article quotes AA as having a success rate of seven to eight percent. Good luck applying conventional statistics to 12-step programs. Anyone who has spent any amount of time hanging around addicts knows that someone trying to get clean or sober or cease any type of compulsive behavior, such as overeating or gambling, can try and fail 365 times in one year alone. If each time counts as a failure, then the statistics would be royally skewed.

Rip-off rehab

The Atlantic article tells the story of an attorney, J. G., who started drinking at 15, and sought help for his alcoholism after he had established his career, "He spent a month at a center where the treatment consisted of little more than attending Alcoholics Anonymous meetings."

J. G.'s rehab was a rip-off. The 2015 documentary *The Business of Recovery* documents the abundance of flawed rehab facilities throughout the US.

Offering only a spiritual remedy to a complex, insidious, and potentially terminal affliction would be akin to firing every medical doctor in every hospital and replacing them with shamans, ministers, and priests.

Addiction is complex because it often masks other issues, such as mental illness, learning differences, post-traumatic stress disorder, poverty, toxic family or marital dynamics, consequences from a lack of nurturing or lack of effective education, and disastrous career choices.

Neurobiology

Except behind the walls of most rehabs, it is no secret that neurobiology often plays a role in addiction—some of us are wired to respond dramatically to various drugs such as stimulants, opiates, and sugar. *The Atlantic* article points out that countries such as Finland routinely assess neurobiological factors in their addiction treatment facilities.

The Sober Truth: Debunking the Bad Science Behind 12-Step Programs and the Rehab Industry by Lance Dodes, MD and Zachary Dodes promotes psychodynamic psychotherapy and dismisses the relationship between neurobiology and addiction.

The New York Times May 5, 2014 article, "Taking Aim at 12-Step Programs" by Richard A. Friedman MD reviews *The Sober Truth*. Quoting Dr. Friedman's 2014 *New York Times* article as to why *The Sober Truth's* premise makes no sense, "This simplistic and unitary model for addiction ignores much of clinical reality: drug abuse driven by novelty and sensation-seeking, which is typical of adolescents; and the high prevalence of substance abuse in patients with major depression and anxiety disorders, most likely a result of efforts to self-medicate."

> *"This simplistic and unitary model for addiction ignores much of clinical reality: drug abuse driven by novelty and sensation-seeking, which is typical of adolescents; and the high prevalence of substance abuse in patients with major depression and anxiety disorders, most likely a result of efforts to self-medicate."*

Responsible rehab

Whatever brain genetics make someone more likely to be an addict, substances such as opiates further disrupt brain function and create overpowering cravings. Effective rehabs should offer addicts a systematic approach for rewiring their thought patterns so that they don't crave their fix and should teach addicts how to develop positive habits to counteract occasional cravings. This could involve personality tests and interest surveys, goal setting, and working with addiction specialists, life coaches, and vocational counselors.

You have to want something more than getting high, and you have to build support systems and take inventory of every individual in your life and every aspect of yourself.

Change is tough. (Regarding changing bad habits or adopting good habits, I would highly recommend reading *Atomic Habits* by James Clear.)

Working a program

Attending 12-step meetings can be inspirational, boring, annoying, or a waste of time. However, those motivated to "work a 12-step program" can learn effective life skills for free such as goal setting, practicing gratitude, introspection, accountability, and building a supportive network. For example, practicing gratitude functions somewhat like cognitive behavioral therapy.

12-step programs are free

Addiction is often the result of a tangled web of adversities and challenges, but our mental health system is its own tangled web. Although 12-step programs are often not enough to address every aspect that led someone to addiction, they are free and accessible.

Higher power

J.G. mastered the art of blame that is essential for every addict. He blamed AA for his relapses. J.G. says it was this message—that there are no small missteps, and one drink might as well be 100—that set him on a cycle of bingeing and abstinence.

The use of the word God also hung up J.G. He must moonlight splitting hairs.

The concept of God baffles me too. However, I do understand the simple concept of a higher power—there is something out there more important than myself.

I do believe in the spiritual energy of the universe that is manifested in nature. The ocean. The sky.

Related links

Many others were taken aback by *The Atlantic* article. Here are a few related links:

- Sarah A. Benton, MS, LMHC, "Irrationality of AA? A critique of the article," May 5, 2015, PsychologyToday.com.

- Katie MacBride, "The Irrationality of The Atlantic's piece on AA," April 3, 2015, Addiction.com.

- Joseph Nowinski, PhD, *If You Work It, It Works!: The Science Behind 12-Step Recovery*, (Hazelden, 2015)

- Tommy Rosen, "Spirituality vs. Science? A Rebuttal to The Atlantic Article, 'The Irrationality of Alcoholics Anonymous," March 20, 2015, *Huffington Post.*

- Jesse Singal, "Why Alcoholics Anonymous Works," March 17, 2015, TheCut.com.

CHAPTER 46

Q&A Interview With Dr. Ted Zeff

Are You Highly Sensitive?

Ted Zeff, PhD author of *The Power of Sensitivity: Success Stories by Highly Sensitive People Thriving in a Non-sensitive World.*

Q: Could you explain the HSP trait?

A: It is not due to something unusual about your eyes, nose, skin, taste buds, or ears. It's that you process sensory information more carefully. It's how your nervous system processes the information coming in. When the HSPs were looking at different pictures, different parts of the brain would light up. There are neurological differences in the way you process energy.

Q: What are the advantages of being a highly sensitive person (HSP) also known as the sensory sensitivity processing trait?

A: There are a lot of wonderful aspects to being an HSP, such as being sensitive to your environment, animals, innovation, and ideas. HSPs tend to be very, very creative, conscientious, and loyal. HSPs notice potential danger. They are natural counselors and share a love for humanity.

When they are not overwhelmed, they experience love and joy more deeply, if raised by parents and have teachers who appreciate their sensitivity.

Q: Why do negative experiences in childhood affect HSPs so much?

A: What studies show is that if you are a highly sensitive person and you had a bad childhood, you will be more affected by your childhood experience than someone who is not highly sensitive.

Research by Dr. Elaine Aron indicated that non-sensitive adults with troubled childhoods did not show nearly as much depression and anxiety as sensitive adults who experienced similar childhood trauma. However, highly sensitive people who had healthy childhoods are as emotionally well-adjusted as their non-HSPs counterparts.

Q: Does being highly sensitive translate into operating in a constant state of overstimulation?

A: it is so important to create an environment that you are not in a constant state of overstimulation. If you have a job where you're commuting, the job is tense, the family situation is high pressure, you could be in a state of overstimulation. The whole key is putting yourself in an environment that is peaceful.

CHAPTER 47

Temperament, Trauma, and Sensitivity

Some compelling research addresses the impact of childhood trauma and the role temperament and environment play.

"The Adverse Childhood Experiences (ACE) Study"

The 1998 ACE Study was published in the *American Journal of Preventive Medicine*. It assessed data from thousands of patients and came up with a system for categorizing and measuring the impact of various kinds of childhood trauma on all aspects of health, including mental health.

"How childhood trauma affects health across a lifetime"

Dr. Nadine Burke Harris's 2014 TED Talk references recent research that further explores and confirms what the ACE study concluded.

Harris points out that for a person with an ACE score of four or more, the likelihood of depression is four and a half times higher and for suicidality 12 times higher.

In her TED Talk, Dr. Harris says, "We now understand better than we ever have before how exposure to early adversity affects the developing brains and bodies of children. It affects areas like the nucleus accumbens, the pleasure and reward center of the brain that is implicated in substance dependence.

"It inhibits the prefrontal cortex, which is necessary for impulse control and executive function, a critical area for learning. And on MRI scans, we see measurable differences in the amygdala, the brain's fear response center.

"So, there are real neurologic reasons why folks exposed to high doses of adversity are more likely to engage in high-risk behavior, and that's important to know. "

"So, there are real neurologic reasons why folks exposed to high doses of adversity are more likely to engage in high-risk behavior, and that's important to know. "

"Dandelions, tulips and orchids: evidence for the existence of low-sensitive, medium-sensitive and high-sensitive individuals"

This study published in 2018 *Translational Psychiatry* explained that different innate temperaments react differently to environmental stressors.

"According to empirical studies and recent theories, people differ substantially in their reactivity or sensitivity to environmental influences with some being generally more affected than others. More sensitive individuals have been described as orchids and less-sensitive ones as dandelions."

"We also detected a third group (40%) characterized by medium sensitivity, which we refer to as tulips in keeping with the flower metaphor."

"Elevated empathy in adults following childhood trauma"

This study published in the medical journal *PLOS ONE* in 2018 concluded that although experiencing childhood trauma can lead to increased vulnerability to depression and addiction, it can also lead to greater empathy.

"These findings suggest that the experience of a childhood trauma increases a person's ability to take the perspective of another and to understand their mental and emotional states and that this impact is long-standing."

Empaths experience music more deeply

The study "Neurophysiological effects of trait empathy in music listening" was published in *Frontiers in Behavioral Neuroscience* in 2018. It used functional magnetic resonance imaging (fMRI) to explore how highly sensitive individuals who more readily experience the emotions of others experience music more profoundly.

"Our study offers novel evidence that neural circuitry involved in trait empathy is active to a greater degree in empathic individuals during perception of both simple musical tones and full musical excerpts."

The study found that highly sensitive, empathetic individuals experience music in the brain regions for reward, social awareness, and regulation of social emotions.

PART FIVE

Insight

"Be who you are and don't allow anyone to affect the confidence you have in your individuality."

–Demi Lovato

CHAPTER 48

Great Recession, Shame, and Relapse

September 2008

It was late in the afternoon when I met Shane, a mystic, and his camerawoman at the rollerblade rental booth in Santa Monica. I was there for my video holo-therapy session, which involved filming me as I rollerbladed in order to analyze my movement.

The camerawoman began filming me as soon as I started coaxing my feet into the rollerblades.

As I skated through the empty section of the vast parking lot adjacent to the bike path and not far from the endless beach, Shane gave me feedback, "You're moving up from one of your shoulders. You have consciousness focused really high. You want to be moving from your second chakra."

He directed my movement through the parking lot. His soft voice was devoid of emotion as he prompted me, "Get in your core, and let your feet feel the ground and direct you, rather than being in your head and thinking about your feet."

It took me several trips back and forth to relax enough to get in my core. Ballet is all about the core, so I knew what he was talking about. He added, "When you are in your core and in your center, your whole life gets a lot easier."

He commented that my female energy, intuition, was much stronger than my male energy, rational thought. And he also made me aware of my hands—energy had to flow through them in order to be open to the energy of the universe.

His goal was to teach individuals how to become centered and move through life present and "in their bodies" as opposed to "in their heads" and constantly replaying the myths (pre-conceived, deep-rooted ideas) they have developed through the years and keep reliving. He believed that skating regularly helped keep you out of your head and your mythology.

I looked tentative on the video. After reviewing the entire video with me, Shane said, "I don't think there is anything wrong with you. I think your bipolar disorder is a learned behavior." At the time, the remark confused me, but I didn't take it too seriously.

However, that remark became a time bomb.

His analysis made me more aware of my body language and the body language of others. Just as smiling can make you feel better, so can walking more confidently.

"It has nothing to do with your work. Please know that. Between the merger and the continued slowdown, we have to reduce our staff," my manager said to me.

Six weeks earlier I had received an excellent review and a small raise. I had survived the first round of layoffs a few months earlier and didn't expect another round to happen so suddenly.

My skating session had taken place two days earlier, which made the bad news even more jarring.

Because I had arranged to leave a little early that day, a Friday, to meet with a refrigerator repairman, I only had enough time to gather my few belongings together before heading out the door. Leaving without saying anything to any of my co-workers made the experience all the more unreal.

While the repairman diagnosed the refrigerator, I calculated the price of the food we had lost while it had gone down. Keith and I had recently separated, which made the layoff seem all the more painful. As a mother, I craved security. I wanted to know that I could provide for my children.

Less than two weeks later I was headed for an interview in Century City for a similar job, writing proposals for a company with national name recognition. One of the national account managers with whom I had worked had recommended me. Wary of the commute, during the phone interview I had inquired about a partial telecommute and had been assured it could be arranged. Working a couple of days from home would make the commute somewhat manageable.

The job I had left had only been 10 miles from home, and I could take streets if necessary. I worked from 7 a.m. to 4 p.m. My commute took around 15 minutes in the morning and 20 to 25 minutes to get home. Most importantly, if I needed to stay late, the length of my commute did not increase exponentially. The proximity gave me the ability to occasionally travel to and from home mid-day to volunteer at school events and then simply make up the time.

The Century City parking structure was the size of a small theme park. To get into the upper floors of the massive office building, one had to navigate two sets of elevators.

Before the interview, I had the opportunity to chat with some of my potential co-workers. One of them admitted, "I usually get on the road about 5 a.m. to beat traffic."

A few days later, I received a phone call from the company's Human Resources department. The representative sounded upbeat and said, "They'd like to meet with you again, but they changed their mind about the partial telecommute."

My heart sank. I instantly knew that I could never survive the horrific traffic that translated into grueling commutes, zero ability to predict when I would arrive home, and being locked into getting up before 5 a.m. every weekday morning.

I scored another interview for a proposal writer. This job was in the same town I lived in, Long Beach. I was pumped. The interview started off on a good note when the manager interviewing me revealed that he was a fellow graduate of Cal State Long Beach. Then he began talking and never stopped.

I did my best to nod my head and say "Sure," as he kept talking. "In addition to proposal writing, your responsibilities would include cataloging and reviewing and evaluating all potential proposals," he said.

He had just finished describing what my manager, myself, and the other proposal writer had done at my prior job.

"You'll have a company phone and laptop for the times you need to work off-site."

He put in a call to another proposal writer back east. It was three hours later, 7:30 at night, in his time zone. This proposal writer seemed desperate to find a replacement for himself, or perhaps I was supposed to report to him.

After he had shown me around the premises, he took me into his office and continued his monologue. The highlight was, "Sasha, I think you could do this job. But for the first two years, you'd be cargo."

He went on to further explain that the training they would provide was so valuable, they would be carrying me for the first two years.

His lecture made me realize that what he termed flexibility really meant that I could leave after a full day's work, pick up my kids, maybe even make dinner, and then get back to work again until it was time to go to sleep.

"Thank you for taking the time to interview me," I said.

"If you have any further questions, please get back to me. We're definitely interested."

I couldn't exit the building fast enough.

I had been laid off at the end of September 2008. My two interviews had been in October, and then everything slowed in mid-November and never picked up. 2009 was the height of the Great Recession.

Day-to-day substitute teaching did not pay much, because of the school holidays, half-day assignments, and days without assignments, but I had done it before, and it was my fall back. It was also meaningful work. However, by the time I got laid off, the economy was so bad the substitute slots had been more than filled. I imagined that some of the slots had been filled by desperate individuals who never expected to substitute teach.

I was beginning to worry. A lot.

CHAPTER 49

Performing Stand-up

January 2009

Friday nights in downtown Long Beach, Coffee Haven hosted a killer Open Mic. I tried to make it there a couple of times a month. Because it was a coffee shop, it was all ages. Often, I would bring my children, if Keith wasn't able to watch them.

My new best friend, Zoe, a fellow single mom, loved attending my Open Mics and occasional comedy shows. Zoe had introduced me to Shane. She credited Shane with transforming her life and would often say to me, "You need to work more with Shane. I don't understand why you're not a CEO or some kind of millionaire." It was easy to write jokes about Zoe.

My New Age friend Zoe and I have a lot in common. We're both single moms.

Her ex-husband is a rock star. My fantasy lover is a rock star.

One Friday night in December my children weren't there, and I opened with the following bit.

I'm getting divorced for the third time. From the same man.

How do you flunk divorce? Run out of the retainer.

Mixed marriages don't work. Creative. Non-creative. "You are just too weird."

I was actually getting divorced for the second time from the same man, but the third time sounded better.

After my set, another comic approached me with a puzzled look on his face and asked, "Did you get remarried again? Did you get presents again?"

We chatted long enough for me to learn his name was Malik, he was new to stand-up, not terribly serious about it, and recently unemployed. Malik was mixed race, almost six feet tall, muscular, but not overly, and walked with a spring in his step. Other than his striking looks, he didn't leave much of an impression on me.

I don't remember the details except that he did contact me with comedy questions, and we ended up on a date.

Stand-up comedy is easily accessible in Long Beach and Los Angeles. Since my writer's conference debut, I had performed in a number of stage shows in the Greater LA Area, but preparing for the longer, more polished sets took away from the little time I carved out of my schedule to write.

I have more than an hour's worth of material, but without a good deal of practice, I can't perform more than 10 minutes. However, performing stand-up comedy once or twice a month at Open Mics became one of my best ways to cope with stress. It put me in touch with the creative part of myself, satisfied my need for thrills, and enabled me to hang out with other creatives.

When Malik offered me a joint a couple of months into our affair, it should have been my cue to exit. While we had been getting to know each other, he had assured me that getting high was something in his past.

It's not something I can be around often. It's one of my non-negotiables along with making sure I get at least seven hours of sleep a night. Although smoking weed never caused any of my episodes, it certainly intensified them and helped tip them from heading towards mania to no way to reverse course into full-blown mania, paranoia, and delusions. The high-level anxiety, agitation, and restlessness of hypomania are what made me seek out marijuana. But once I started getting high, I could not stop for weeks. By then, I had achieved full-blown mania.

I had put down drugs, alcohol, and overeating. I wasn't a sex addict, but when I fell into a relationship in which the sex was phenomenal… the sex became like a drug. Perhaps even more so, because I could only see Malik once a week.

In preparing for a follow-up all-day training hosted by Shane, I weaned myself off of my medication. On the day of the event, all I remember is getting hopelessly lost finding the Santa Monica hotel. My late arrival, not to mention my full-blown panic attack that had escalated to shaking and sobbing, was met with frowns, and the greeter at the door turned me away.

Thus, began my last relapse in March 2009, which shook me to my core.

"You're smoking?" Malik exclaimed as his eyebrows raised. Even though he was a smoker, he seemed shocked to witness me smoking a cigarette.

I hadn't had a cigarette in years. I knew cigarettes were bad for the heart and lungs and didn't intend to smoke for long, but being unemployed was getting to me, and now, too, the uncertainty of my relationship with him. Nicotine helped me concentrate, and it relaxed me.

Within a couple of weeks, I had worked my way up to a pack of cigarettes a day.

I had been a weekend smoker from age 12 until I quit at 13. I started smoking again, intermittently, at 19, and sometimes went for years without smoking. Never before though had I smoked a pack of cigarettes a day. My habit had mostly been a pack a week or less and occasionally two packs a week.

When I smoked only one to three cigarettes a day, the nicotine instantly overtook me and enabled me to concentrate intensely for several hours thereafter.

The uncertainty of being unemployed made me anxious, and I could not stand feeling anxious. Although I had given up drugs, alcohol, and compulsive overeating, I didn't see that, by smoking, I was trading addictions once again.

I attribute becoming a smoker to my inability to handle uncomfortable feelings and insecurity—the core of addiction.

The average person is not risking mania from smoking, but nicotine is a stimulant. Smoking a pack of cigarettes a day turned out to be akin to snorting crystal meth for me. At the time, I did not see smoking cigarettes as a threat to my mental health. In hindsight, I can see that a high amount of nicotine was a significant factor in my relapse.

I can't blame Shane for not believing in mental illness, because he's certainly not alone. Shane didn't cause my relapse. Shame caused my relapse.

Although I had accepted my diagnosis many years before and had gone to great lengths to learn everything I could about my illness and to modify my lifestyle to increase my chances of avoiding relapse, I still felt tremendous shame.

Shame made me want to believe I could be cured and done with it and not need medication.

I also experienced shame from having been the victim of child abuse. I remember being about five years old when a woman on the sidewalk in our Washington Heights neighborhood confronted my grandmother. She was horrified at how my grandmother was berating me and screaming orders at me. I had felt so ashamed.

In high school, I would sometimes feel like white trash, because I was getting beaten up behind closed doors.

I had replayed the illogic of the childhood dynamic I had played out with my father by subconsciously seeking approval from Shane, someone to whom I looked up to and regarded as more educated, more accomplished, and more worthy than myself. Was I doomed to repeat this dynamic again and again?

CHAPTER 50

Another Miracle

April 2009

I heard a knock on the door. I got up from sorting children's clothing and my freelance writing files and opened the door to reveal a weary-looking middle-aged woman.

In a soft voice, she identified herself as being with the Department of Children and Family Services (DCFS). She explained that she needed to interview me and then needed to interview my son and my daughter who were at school. As I answered her questions, she took notes. "May I look around?" she asked. In a state of semi-shock, I gave her a tour of the house.

A recent incident replayed in my mind. I had been smoking a cigarette in my car with the windows rolled up. When I rolled them down to air out the car before picking up my children, a fellow parent, a father, had given me an odd look in the elementary school parking lot. I had felt offended. Self-conscious about my newly-bleached platinum blonde short hair, I had blurted out, "You look like you work for the government."

His entire face had scowled. I waited until he left before entering the building to sign out my children. The after-school program supervisor pulled me aside and told me he had asked her to call the police, but her response had been, "But she didn't do anything."

I guessed that father called DCFS, but the day the DCFS worker showed up I thought it would all turn out to be a misunderstanding. I had never neglected or abused my children.

Weeks later I was shown the report from that first day, and the DCFS worker had categorized the house as disorganized and made other negative statements. She had not been impressed with my sorting efforts. No one has ever nominated me for Ms. Housekeeper USA, but one of my part-time jobs in college had been cleaning houses, and I am generally tidy.

The first hearing took place within two weeks. The judge ruled that I could only see my children in the presence of a DCFS-approved monitor. I was told that there would be another hearing in six months in which I could permanently lose custody of my children.

After hearing the verdict, I remember heading to a secluded spot outside the courthouse and sobbing so hard that I howled.

My DCFS caseworker gave me a long list of assignments, such as anger management classes, parenting classes, drug testing, and more that I needed to complete in order to have a chance at regaining custody.

I had been working steps in a different 12-step program that focused on the dynamics of relationships, but once the shock had worn off, I shifted my focus to NA and got a new sponsor. NA was more intense, which is what I needed. Other moms who had passed through the rooms had lost and regained custody of their children, which gave me hope.

One of the tenets of all 12-step programs is to own your part in any and every situation and to focus on those actions for which you have control, your own actions. Let go of blame. Shift focus from problems to potential solutions. Then pray for acceptance, and let go of attachment to outcomes.

It was painful to imagine my children in foster care as a potential outcome. I had to stop doing that. I had to focus on doing what was being asked of me by DCFS, working with my new sponsor, getting the most I could out of my training program, and continuing to get more adept at my job search. Regarding the job search, letting go of attachment to potential outcomes was akin to trying not to pick at a scab on your knee. However, objectivity made the process more like playing a game than contemplating one's remaining destiny.

"Just do the next right thing," is a 12-step slogan that helps with focus. I get it. I do it, but I still tend toward panic at times. In a way, depression is a sense of overwhelming, immobilizing panic.

> What is my part?
> How do I start?
> Bye, bye regret.

During one of my weekly monitored visits, my DCFS caseworker stood off to the side of the summer day camp outdoor play area. He never said much, but his brows were always knit together as if he were evaluating my every word and gesture.

My 10-year-old son had trouble making eye contact with me. Was this the same child who, as a first-grader, had proudly admitted that he had beaten a fifth-grader at tetherball... who, as a third-grader, was overjoyed when he hit a grand slam his first season playing baseball?

My five-year-old daughter looked around as if scoping out the area. Something seemed different, but I couldn't figure out what.

My first bout of extended unemployment as a mom, and, ironically, I was being forced to clean out my savings to pay for summer daycare.

Some days I felt as if I were going to explode from the emotional pain.

As a motherless child, I had experienced the unspeakable. My worst fear, leaving my children motherless, was being realized.

July 2009

I knew Tracy from the local comedy circuit. She was a pharmaceutical rep but also produced a one-hour weekly radio show. The owner of Coffee Haven had purchased a 30-minute slot for comics. He had left it to Andy, one of the regulars who made a living producing comedy shows, to book the comedians. Andy had booked several comedians, including me.

Tracy's own health woes involved an overactive thyroid. She claimed her ex-boyfriend was entering her house and rearranging things and other odd occurrences. Her story didn't exactly add up, but she lived close by and didn't mind going to listen to local live music with me. On the Fourth of July, she took me to her temple in Long Beach for some sort of spiritual ceremony. All I remember is that we met outdoors. Some meditation and chanting were involved. Not too much talking. I went home feeling relaxed.

The next morning, I woke up hovering above myself and objectively evaluating my behavior for the last three months. Malik had drifted away, but the moment he had smoked a joint in front of me, I should have walked out the door. Since moving downtown, I had kept some sketchy company. This horrified me. Suddenly, I realized I had been manic.

Suddenly, I no longer was.

Once the realization sunk in that I had not been acting like myself, I struggled with feelings of dread and shame. The only way I survived was by leaning on my spiritual discipline, which enabled me to trust, to let go, and to focus on positive things, such as the Saturday evening prayer group held at the church near the apartment I was now renting.

September 2009

All my time spent at the Unemployment Insurance program's Workforce Development Center paid off in a minor miracle. I received a voucher to attend a full-time training program related to my field. After checking out three programs on their list of approved programs, I chose the New Horizons training program for website-related software applications (Dreamweaver, Photoshop, InDesign, and Illustrator) that was housed in a modern facility only 30 minutes away and adjacent to Angel Stadium.

November 2009

While I was in the midst of an online job search, my cellphone began to ring. The caller identified herself as the supervising attorney at the law firm the court had assigned to me and then said, "Your attorney resigned. Since your hearing is less than a week away, I need to take over your case."

At a loss for words, I simply said, "Thank you."

"You have fulfilled everything they asked of you. Why is your DCFS caseworker still recommending monitored visits?"

"I don't know. It didn't make sense to me either."

"I need them to change that recommendation," she said before hanging up.

My hearing was scheduled for Monday, November 9, 2009. Close to 9 p.m. on the Friday before, my new attorney called and said, "It took a while, but I got your caseworker to change the recommendation."

My previous attorney, the one who had resigned, had barely said anything to me. He would never have worked overtime to fight for my children and me.

It was truly a miracle that he had resigned, and I had ended up with a powerhouse attorney.

Monday, the hearing went like clockwork and I regained custody. The judge commended me for all of my hard work. It didn't hurt that Keith and I had gotten back together in September. With the way things had been going with DCFS, I had been petrified that my children would end up in foster care. I had taken it as a sign from the universe to give the marriage one more chance to prevent that outcome.

Although I never neglected or abused my children, in the spring of 2009, for a few months, I hadn't been myself. I had been agitated, mildly paranoid, and nearly incapable of getting anywhere on time. I stepped back to figure out why it had happened.

Aside from smoking a pack of cigarettes a day and abandoning medication, I had allowed friends into my life who were critical of the need for treatment for addiction and mental illness. These friends believed both were simply a result of being weak-willed and all one needed to do was to "grow up." For example, I had allowed my New Age friend Zoe to become an insidious negative influence. I also realized that creatives are in the minority and that I needed to have some friends or acquaintances who also had the discipline to pursue creative projects.

Attending training full-time and then working part-time a few months at the Gap during the extended Christmas season helped energize me for my job search, and I landed an excellent technical writing job in April 2010.

For six months, I put aside volunteering, writing, comedy, and everything else outside of my new job aside from taking care of my children every day and attending a 12-step meeting at least once a week.

However, by the end of the six months, it was clear to me that the dynamic that had threatened our marriage before had returned.

CHAPTER 51

Addicted to Approval

2012

"Please, can we stop by?" my son asked. He and his friend had just finished playing a Sunday baseball game within two miles of my father's home. We hadn't visited there in more than three years. Although the 75-mile drive to their home can take three to four hours in traffic, we hadn't visited, because my stepmother had said to me, "You are dead to me," right after my last episode in 2009.

My son's teammate and his father, my daughter, my son, and I piled into my red Toyota Matrix for the five-minute drive to my father's suburban five-bedroom house.

My father answered the door and escorted us into the living room. His wife was there along with a woman I had never seen before who appeared to be about my stepmother's age and vaguely European.

"This is my friend Natalia. She is visiting from Europe. I haven't seen her since medical school," my stepmother said by way of introduction.

They began speaking in their native language, which I could still understand, and they were diagnosing me. They shook their heads in unison as if horrified at my mental condition. According to them, I was headed toward mania.

I was talking a little fast, but I was making sense. I was nervous. My stepmother made me very nervous. Or rather, I let her make me nervous.

I had been researching bipolar disorder for almost 20 years and had the diagnostic criteria memorized. According to the Mayo Clinic's website, mania and hypomania include three or more of the following symptoms:

- Abnormally upbeat, jumpy, or wired

- Increased activity, energy, or agitation

- An exaggerated sense of well-being and self-confidence (euphoria)

- Decreased need for sleep

- Unusual talkativeness

- Racing thoughts

- Distractibility

- Impaired judgment resulting in reckless behavior, such as excessive gambling, overspending, taking sexual risks, or making foolish investments

In my head, I defended myself by reciting all the things I would love to say to her, but because she was agitated and prejudiced against me, there would have been no point.

I am responsible for every area of my life. I work hard at my technical writing job. I take care of my children almost all on my own and make a point to network with other devoted parents. I volunteer in the community. I sleep, exercise, eat well, research,

*and write feature articles regarding bipolar disorder for a mental
health magazine with high editorial standards.*

I didn't meet any of the criteria for mania or hypomania,
yet their judgment rattled me.

During the exchange, my father had been outside with
my son, my son's friend, and the father of my son's friend.
My daughter had been wandering around the ground floor
of the large two-story home. It was a long drive home, and
everyone was ready to go.

"I'm sorry I disturbed your peace," I said to my stepmother
as we prepared to leave. Our visit had lasted less than half
an hour.

As soon as the five of us piled into my Toyota Matrix, my
daughter asked, "Why does she hate you so much?"

"She doesn't hate me. She was upset." As soon as I said
that, I thought to myself, *I should have answered I don't know.*

The visit must have been strange for my eight-year-old
daughter. My stepmother had doted on Laura from the time
she was six months old until the time she was five years old and
my stepmother had stopped talking to me and my children.
Laura hadn't seen her in three years. After such a long break,
it must have been jarring for her to see the woman who had
bounced her around, made her laugh, taken her clothes shopping, and treated her to salon haircuts behaving so differently.

My son had not met my stepmother until he was five years
old, because my stepmother had also refused to talk to me
from 1993 until 2003 as punishment for my manic episode
in 1993. However, even though my grandmother had been 80
years old when Patrick was born, she had doted on him during
his preschool years. One or two days a week, she would pick
Patrick up from preschool and take him to Big Lots or to the
park and then home for homemade lemon bars, pot roast, or
whatever else she had cooked.

The next day it hit me. Why should I care what this woman
thought of me? Why was I always trying to be friends with her?

She was highly accomplished in her profession, an amazing cook, and oozed fashion flair, but why was I still so in awe of her when she had treated me so cruelly.

For years, I had been seeking her approval. That was on me. I realized I needed to let go of seeking her approval.

Laura

Look and you'll see

My hair is a yellow river
My eyes watching like an eagle

My arms are looking for a friend
My heart is filled with funniness

I'm the one you could play with
I never will not do my homework

My daughter Laura wrote this poem about herself in elementary school. I bless the teacher who coaxed this poem out of her. At 17, she aspires to be an environmental engineer, not a poet.

Joshua Tree

The slight breeze in the air
The iron-rich landscape
Cactus everywhere you turn

We strut along
No destination in sight
Only the hills to guide us

We are one with the earth

At 21, my son Patrick aspires to be a hydrogeologist, not a poet. He plays the guitar and loves music as much as I do though. I am deeply grateful that Patrick and his girlfriend Aly treat each other with appreciation, affection, and respect.

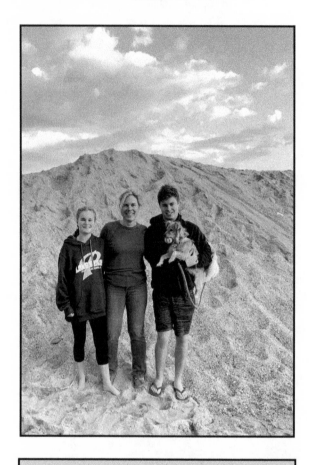

Laura, myself, and Patrick (holding
Charlie) December 31, 2018.

CHAPTER 52

Group Therapy for Codependency

2012

It had taken me 18 months to convince my healthcare provider that I would benefit from treatment for codependency. I had been completely unaware that such treatment existed until a member of one of my 12-step groups detailed her experience with group therapy for codependency.

"You're too healthy," was what I had heard at my intake evaluation with a therapist. The psychiatrist I met with every four months had been skeptical too. Dr. Kandy could no longer be my psychiatrist because Keith had switched our health insurance plan in 2010.

I found my way to my provider's Chemical Dependency Center, CDC, by accident. While at a March 2012 presentation by IWOSC, Independent Writers of Southern California, I met a fellow writer who had worked for my healthcare provider. She told me to call the CDC directly for an intake interview, and they would decide whether I was a candidate for treatment.

During my intake interview with the CDC therapist, an addiction specialist, he cut me off and said, "There's no logic with an addict."

I thought to myself, *This is different.* Other than the year and a half with Sarah, and the intermittent sessions here and there, I had not been in therapy much, but no one had ever interrupted me before.

By the end of the intake interview, I was granted approval to attend group therapy for codependency.

The dynamic of group therapy led by a seasoned addiction specialist provided me with insight that individual therapy could not have. An intellectual understanding is one thing, an emotional understanding another, but, for some, including me, traumatic experiences in one's childhood settle into your very essence. Everyone in the group had a family member or close friend who struggled with addiction.

What anyone else shared is confidential, so I won't elaborate, but sitting in a room and listening to others share similar experiences and then hearing the therapist and participants in the group provide feedback provided a powerful reality check.

It was as if the addicts all had the same playbook. Deny. Deflect. Bolt.

Whereas the 12-step model would be quite different. Step back. Reflect. Adjust.

Watching the therapist interact with the others was far more powerful for me than a one-to-one interaction would have been.

Some things the therapist said imprinted themselves in my brain, such as, "If you wait to feel different, feel better, feel like taking an action before you do take the action, it's not going to happen. You have to take the action and then the feeling will follow." He had explained a basic principle of cognitive behavioral therapy, which I had never before connected to the 12-step slogan, "Act as if."

I separated from Keith in July of 2012. It happened to be Bastille Day.

The payoff from two years of attending group therapy almost every week was feeling as if I was getting to know myself all over again. I also realized that I would always have to be aware of my tendency to please others and to put their needs before my own.

After working through steps in three 12-step programs, making major lifestyle changes, such as abandoning sugar, white flour, binge eating, drugs, and alcohol, successfully managing bipolar disorder for years, and two years of highly effective group therapy, you would think that I would be immune to falling for a middle-aged man with the emotional maturity of a teenager.

CHAPTER 53

Mr. Smooth

2015

I never understood Internet dating. I meet men on the sidewalk. Of course, some of them turn out to be living on the sidewalk.

In summer, at the beach, it's hard to tell. Is he tanning? Is he homeless?

My 95-year-old grandmother died in May 2015. She had been in failing health for months, but her death hit me hard. I clung to the happy memories I had of her, such as her 90th birthday during which my father had held court. After dinner and birthday cake, one of the guests had asked my Uncle Pete, "How many does your RV sleep?"

My father had answered for him, "That depends on their sex." Everyone at the table had laughed.

As the laughter died down, he had added, "If they're women, it sleeps six." More laughter.

"And if they're up to my standard, then it sleeps 12. He can handle a harem." By then, everyone at the table had tears in their eyes from laughing so hard.

When the conversation turned to stand-up comics, my father had performed a version of one of Richard Pryor's bits about visiting an Arizona prison, which had made everyone there howl with laughter.

In addition to his charm, quick wit, and charisma, my father had also been a master at manipulating women with his poor-me-take-care-of-me-I-need-you act.

Who wants to be a cliché? However, as far as daddy issues go, I still had this Pavlovian attraction to charismatic, manipulative men.

The light-hearted account I wrote about my disastrous 2015 love affair with Randy, a.k.a. Mr. Smooth, for the September 5, 2015, *Los Angeles Times* L.A. Affairs column helped provide closure.

L.A. Affairs: How she plans to manifest Mr. Right—and get off the dating merry-go-round for good

Many singles meet their dates on the Internet. I prefer to meet men on the sidewalk. Parking lots, bleachers, In-n-Outs or comedy clubs work too. Maybe I've read too much metaphysics or watched too much OWN, but I believe that I can manifest the right mate by becoming completely clear about the person I am meant to be and the man who should become my mate.

So, one and a half years after separating from my husband of 17 years and the father of my two kids, I made a list of the qualities I desired in a man—passionate about his work, volunteer in the community, a father or step-father, athletic, funny, does not use drugs or drink excessively, and does not smoke.

A month later, I found myself in an Orange County high school parking lot cleaning out my car as I waited for my son's baseball game to begin. Toting a plastic bag full of empty water bottles, snack wrappers, apple cores, and crumpled homework, I asked a man hosting an earthquake preparedness event where I could find a trashcan. By the first pitch, he had my phone number.

Mark met every qualification on my list. A divorced dad, he was close to his 20-something daughter, he loved his job, he was an integral part of his community and the school district for which he worked, he had played high school sports, and he was passionate about his health.

On our fourth date, lunch, he told me an anecdote about a family member that would have enraged most people I know. Mark simply shrugged his shoulders with acceptance and asked me how my daughter's friend liked the fake fish tank he had given her. Mark and I had gone to a New Year's Eve party that included a White Elephant exchange. When my 10-year-old daughter's friend had coveted the gift my daughter had ended up with, he had tracked down another one and bought it for her.

I returned to my office thinking, what a classy gentleman. I found Mark attractive, and I badly wanted to make him my boyfriend, but there was no spark.

Five months after meeting Mark, I met "Randy" in a different parking lot. He had the body of a skier and the voice of a rock star. His 6-foot-tall body was lithe and his hazel eyes sparkled. My list went out the window. We fell into conversation, and he impressed me with his knowledge of music education. For a month, we spoke on the phone several nights a week. I wasn't sure if we were simply becoming friends until he sent me this text, "I must confess that since the first time we met, I have had a strange attraction for you that I am almost afraid to pursue. I said almost."

Three months after our parking lot meeting, we had a midnight date. I have never had a better time.

Still, we were not a perfect fit, and after a few months, Randy moved 80 miles away—another time zone in Southern California traffic. I wouldn't hear from him for days at a time. Instead of changing my status on Facebook to single, I simply let the universe know that I was available.

On a rare night out to see a friend perform stand-up at Bogey's in Redondo Beach, I fell into conversation with Ian, a fellow former New Yorker. He walked me to my car and I couldn't say no to an invitation to walk on the Hermosa Beach Strand and have dinner at The Spot.

In the three weeks before I had a Saturday evening free, I came to enjoy chatting with Ian. It took the sting out of my stop-and-go commute on the 405. A former teacher, Ian asked me lots of questions about my novel and other creative pursuits. His positivity made me realize how critical of me Randy had been, and how easily pheromones tricked me into overlooking his negativity.

One day I had an epiphany—the chemistry I felt with Randy might always be off the charts, but so might his unpredictable behavior. My body said more, but I forced myself to step back and evaluate. Since beginning our affair, my writing had stalled, I was more irritable and absent-minded, and I had stopped performing stand-up.

I debated whether I could get past Ian's being 14 years my junior. He eventually moved out of state.

Meanwhile, I headed back to New York at the end of 2014 for a Christmas vacation, with tentative plans to meet a high school friend. I had always found David attractive, kind, dryly humorous, and slightly silly. I knew he wasn't married but had no idea whether he had a girlfriend.

We hiked the grounds of the Rockefeller Estate, catching up. By the time he kissed me, it felt exciting and familiar at the same time. "I'm glad we got that out of the way," he quipped.

However, our relationship did not make it through the summer. It was such a positive experience though that as far as the universe is concerned, I can only say, "Thank you. Almost perfect."

What wasn't included in the sunny *LA Times* account was that within two weeks of that midnight date, Mr. Smooth flipped a switch. He began alternating recounting his amusing anecdotes with outbursts and insults. Randy had ADHD and dyslexia. At first, I sympathized with him as I had experienced my own learning challenges.

Within two months of that midnight date, I discovered that Mr. Smooth, a man who did not drink, did not use drugs, and did not even smoke cigarettes, was a gambler. I had never met a gambler. I was shocked.

As much as I had come to love him, I couldn't be in a relationship with someone in active addiction and remain intact.

I found out as much as I could about gambling. I discovered that anyone struggling with an addiction to gambling was eligible to receive 10 free therapy sessions through the California Council on Problem Gambling (calpg.org). This had been established as a concession toward allowing legalized gambling in the state of California. Randy did not have health insurance, but he was not interested in the free sessions.

I attended a few meetings of Gam-Anon, the 12-step support group for family and friends of gamblers, and heard about homes being secretly mortgaged away and worse consequences. Ironically, I came across a link between bipolar and gambling as noted in the research study, "Gambling problems in bipolar disorder in the UK: prevalence and distribution" published in the October 2015 issue of *The British Journal of Psychiatry*, "Moderate to severe gambling problems were four times higher in people with bipolar disorder than in the general population and were associated with type 2 disorder."

I had a hard time forgiving myself for falling for Mr. Smooth, someone who had the maturity of a 16-year-old. How could I not have seen through him? I was in group therapy for codependency.

I was not manic. I did not rush into the relationship. I was many years clean, sober, and abstinent from compulsive overeating.

Eventually, I concluded that he had provided an escape from a grueling commute and a challenging job—a job in which I was somewhat a fish out of water. My co-workers chattered about remodels and restaurants while I longed to chatter about rewrites and current events.

At the time, other than my 45-minute lunchtime exercise sessions, I was driving or sitting almost every waking hour seven days a week, and I had my children seven days a week.

Painful lesson—I came to realize that I was much more of a thrill-seeker than I ever imagined. That writing and performing weren't nice-to-haves. They were must-to-haves. Albeit in the small bits I could manage them between working and child-rearing.

My relationship with David had concluded the L.A. Affairs column. David had been affectionate and attentive. I was absolutely attracted to him. However, breaking up with him had been a breakthrough of sorts. No drama. We remained friends. The pain of the uncertainty as to the future of our long-distance relationship was not worth my commitment to it.

I walked away using positive self-talk to recognize my self-worth. *I constantly challenge myself. I juggle two careers. I am a devoted parent. I am as active in the community as possible. And, I make sure to get enough sleep, not go more than one or two days without exercising, and do many other things in order not to jeopardize my health.*

Positive self-talk does not come naturally to me. I had to detach and think of myself as a close friend and what I would tell her.

I reminded myself that for me to devote the energy necessary to a relationship, a love affair, the man has to be sincere about pursuing a relationship too, be committed to his own health, and be willing to challenge himself in his own endeavors.

CHAPTER 54

Piecing Together Clues

2015

One of my father's two brothers, an eye surgeon, was semi-retired. He and his wife traveled frequently, but one fall Friday night in 2015, they were able to make it over for dinner. On the rare occasion I saw this uncle, he almost always brought up my mother and how much he missed her.

We had finished eating salmon, salad, and baked potatoes and were lingering at the table sipping coffee and tea, when my uncle made a startling revelation, "Your father locked your mother out of the house. He had you with him.

"She had to go to the neighbor's and call our mother. That is how I know what happened."

This had happened in the 1960s, long before cellphones. Immediately what came to mind was a story Mor Mor had told me.

"Your mother felt so guilty that she was locked out and couldn't get to you. She had forgotten her keys." Mor Mor had told me that story several times as she had other stories about my mother. Yet she had blocked out that her daughter's husband had angrily locked her out of the house and temporarily held her three-year-old daughter, me, hostage.

My uncle was a credible source. All of a sudden, the few first-hand accounts I had heard through the years of incidents related to events near the end of her life clicked.

My mother's car accident had been mysterious. I had not been allowed to attend the funeral. For several years after her death, I would dream about her. I missed her terribly and replayed my few memories of her like a slideshow in my head.

I remember…

… my mother helping me climb onto a stool, setting me up with utensils, and patiently instructing me as to when to flip the pancake circles the size of my three-year-old fist.

… skipping with her down the sidewalk as she clutched my hand, probably on our way to nowhere special. My mother had a way of turning everyday tasks into adventures.

… my mother saying, "Leftovers taste even better. Never waste food," as she patiently showed me how to place the rest of my tuna sandwich into a plastic container and then into the refrigerator so I could eat it later.

… not feeling sleepy, getting out of bed, tiptoeing down the stairs, quietly sitting down in a roomy upholstered living room chair, and tucking my legs to my side. My mother was folding laundry and did not see me at first. Within a couple of minutes, she caught a glimpse of me and stood up. With her mouth opened wider than I had ever seen it, she groaned, "Ohhh!" Then she chased me back up the stairs. My mother tucked me into my bed and said something to the effect of, "Little girls need their sleep."

My uncle's revelation became a significant clue in the puzzle that was my mother's death. Over the next few days, more pieces of the puzzle ran through my thoughts.

Years before, my ex-stepmother had provided a couple of clues when she and I had reunited in Pennsylvania and spent the weekend together. During one long walk through the woods, she had revealed that my mother had taken a photo of her face with my father's handprint clearly visible in red against her fair skin. My father must have revealed this to her in one of his apology-it-won't-happen-again sessions with her.

More recently, during a phone call, she had revealed that my father had been perplexed as to how my mother could have run into an oil truck going in the other direction on a road she frequently traveled.

Mor Mor had provided another clue. Several times she had reflected about the divorce attorney with whom my mother had consulted and who had said, "Wait until after the child is born. Otherwise, everyone will think the baby is not your husband's."

Having been pregnant with a second child while a working mom, I knew the exhaustion my mother must have experienced. The stress from an abusive partner could only have added to the exhaustion. I remembered what it had been like to live with my father.

The accident had happened in the early morning around 6:30 a.m. My mother had been on her way to turn in grades. There could have been fog.

Out of nowhere, this plausible explanation as to factors that could have contributed to her accident had emerged, exhaustion and possible fog.

I still miss her. I ache for her at times, for her open mind, her open heart, her curiosity, her resourcefulness, and her energy. I especially miss that my children don't have her as a grandmother. From everything I ever learned about her through her college friends and others, she had a magnanimous spirit.

In 2007, one of her college friends sent me a poem about my mother that she had prepared for their 50-year Smith College reunion.

Cynnie, Class of 1957 (excerpted)

A radiant smile was her signature; it accentuated the high color of her Scandinavian complexion and strongly built body intent on adventure, especially in the mountains.

Cynnie was a steadfast friend and an individualist filled with talent and more plans than time.

She was whimsical and charmingly naïve.

When her husband's department chair came to dinner, she served a huge pot of boiled potatoes ("no time to cook").

A little short on French preparation in Geneva, she wore a V-neck black sweater to the tutorial with her professor.

A memory I cherish—Cynnie hanging upside down in a tree on the Amherst campus, choking with laughter, calling out to us to follow.

She was a free spirit.

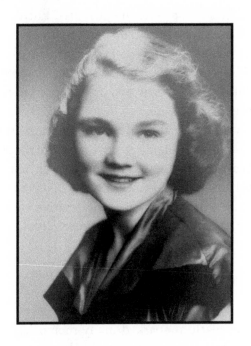

The poem made me cry because it made me realize that I had inherited her whimsical nature and her originality and that those traits had nothing to do with my illness. Although my mother was a college French and Spanish professor, from all accounts she had a keen sense of humor and plenty of flair. Creativity.

When you hear the adjective creative, the first thing that comes to mind is artist, musician, actor, or fashion designer, but creativity applies to far more than the arts. Entrepreneurship, invention, science, marketing, devising innovative solutions to challenges, everyday problem solving, and more benefit from creativity. However, aside from creatives who have achieved celebrity status, creativity is not truly appreciated or understood in American culture.

Research has demonstrated the link between creativity and bipolar. Those who are highly creative are more adept at coming up with ideas, divergent thinking. The trick is figuring out how to constructively deal with the flow of ideas by having an outlet through which to channel the creative energy. If ideas constantly pop up but never go anywhere, that's distracting and exhausting.

My uncle's revelations sparked many memories. In 2005 or 2006, my children were quite young. The four of us had ventured to Newhall, California to visit the family of my Swedish grandmother's brother. Although they only lived 60 miles away, traffic made a weeknight visit impossible and meant that one had to basically devote an entire weekend day for a visit.

After an elegant lunch, we sat down to look at old photos, and I came across one of my mother's father I had never seen before. It had been taken about a year before he died at the age of 67. The bloat was unmistakable. His symmetrical face that I had always classified as boring-handsome was distorted and almost unrecognizable. High blood pressure was what my grandmother had said killed her husband. (Alcoholism can cause high blood pressure.) This photo revealed bloat which was almost certainly from alcohol. I had heard through the years from various relatives that my grandfather, a doctor, had drunk a lot, but never paid that much mind until I saw that photo. By then, I had encountered alcoholics bloated from years of drinking.

His wife, my grandmother, had never mentioned his drinking or that he died from alcoholism, just as she had been in denial of my father's abuse of her daughter and of me. How does that denial make me feel now?

I can still remember the anguish and confusion and aloneness I felt as a child enduring the abuse without anyone to turn to. Sometimes, as a child, I felt as if I were around robots that weren't quite human.

But now, I try to put myself in her shoes. She adored her husband, and it would have been nearly impossible to leave him in those times. I don't understand why or how she overlooked my father's abuse, but she was kind and loving to me when I was a child.

By college, I wondered if my mother had committed suicide because silence and mystery surrounded her death. I now think the hush hush was because of the inability of any of my relatives to acknowledge the burgeoning domestic violence.

From what I now know of domestic violence, usually, the only way to leave is to secretly run away while the abuser is elsewhere. It sounds as if my mother was trying to line everything up or, perhaps, still trying to work things out. In the 1960s there wasn't as much discussion about the profile of a domestic abuser, and the stigma of divorce was much stronger.

I had always thought that what pushed my father over the edge was losing his wife and soon-to-be second child. When those clues came together to paint a picture of a controlling, jealous, and abusive spouse, that theory blew up.

My childhood was confusing. Despite the violence, trauma, and the experience of often being left on my own as early as nine years old, my father did many positive things as a parent.

My father nurtured my self-sufficiency. I was cooking by the age of nine and able to clean an entire house by the age of 12. He fostered my creativity by restricting my television viewing and exposing me to art lessons, music lessons, and foreign language instruction.

I remember a frequent conversation we used to have, "Dad, I'm bored."

"No, you're boring. If you can't find a way to entertain yourself, then, you are boring."

I still don't understand my father's moods or his selective memory, but I do enjoy watching him enjoy my children on the rare occasions he visits with them. The twisted bond that kept me dependent on his approval has been broken, and for that I am grateful.

The beauty of having worked the 12 steps several times is that I tend not to see black and white, but shades of gray. I now own my part of my relationship with my father. It is my choice as to whether to have a relationship with him and my responsibility to establish boundaries.

Although I forgave his abuse many years ago, the subtle ways in which it affected my self-image have posed a challenge.

CHAPTER 55

Potlucks

2016

The lure of sugar has never entirely gone away. After years of banning chocolate from my repertoire, I discovered dark chocolate—not the supermarket dark chocolate, the real thing, 85 percent cacao—so bitter that it is impossible to eat more than four tiny squares. It has an invigorating scent akin to strong coffee. My safe chocolate fix calms me just a little, thrills me just a little, and even somewhat curbs my appetite.

Potlucks at my workplace posed a sugar dilemma, and it didn't take much to get a potluck on the calendar. A full moon. A new hire. A team member's birthday. Another team member's half-birthday.

Every potluck, a co-worker never failed to hand me a paper plate bearing some sugar-infused baked item. "Have a brownie," had replaced, "How are you?"

"No thank you," I would respond and then quickly change the subject by predicting the following day's weather.

But the offers would keep coming. After the third offer of yet another goodie, generally homemade 7-Up cake, I would blurt, "I don't eat sugar. I have sugar sensitivity."

I might as well have confessed to being in a cult. This admission, made at almost every work event marked by sugar confections was always met with a puzzled glance. Despite the diversity and inclusion training we received, turning down Chocolate Bundt Cake proved to be more diversity than my department could handle.

Life would have been much easier if I had lied and said I was diabetic. But then how could I tell my children to value honesty, if their mom lies for convenience?

Fall 2016, we had a two-month stretch of almost daily themed spreads of edibles that culminated in October with Customer Service Week. That week, there was an array of goodies every day beautifully arranged on lace doilies on top of a wide, low filing cabinet less than three feet from my cubicle.

I made it through almost the entire two months, but by Wednesday of Customer Service Week, every 30 minutes or so, I would tiptoe the five steps to the cabinet and fill my tiny, shiny paper dessert plate with brownies. When they ran out, chocolate chip cookies did the trick.

Thursday the only item that called out to me was light, airy, not-too-sweet cinnamon coffee cake from Panera Bread. Unfortunately, it did not call out to anyone else. By the time I headed home, I had finished the entire coffee cake piece by piece.

Were 14 years of abstinence down the drain? That question haunted me for days until I finally realized that however successfully I had evolved, I would never have enough resolve to sit next to my drug of choice for nine hours a day week after week and be able to resist.

CHAPTER 56

Three Miles an Hour

2017

Rush hour commuting is not driving. It is a neurological assault. And in Southern California, rush hour can begin at sunrise and not end until past sunset. I began commuting in April 2010, and it became my biggest health stressor.

Commuting to Irvine from Long Beach involves surviving the long stretch past the Orange County airport where traffic slows to three miles per hour. I can *walk* faster than three miles an hour. A typical day...

While driving during rush hour, my eyes dart everywhere. You can never be too alert in traffic that, without warning, goes from 50 miles per hour to zero miles per hour. Every time a car cuts in and takes away the safety zone I create around my vehicle, I startle.

I witness dented, mangled cars off to the side of the freeway and picture blood and bones poking through flesh as I speculate about the extent of passenger injuries.

While my car crawls its way home, my thoughts are consumed with attempting to figure out how I can pull off showing up at all the places I am supposed to after work.

When I finally make it home, my gait is unsteady as I exit my car. I can feel myself vibrating. My brain seems stuck. The neighbors must think I overdid Happy Hour, but, no, I have just survived the 405 Freeway.

"What's for dinner," my daughter asks as I stumble through the doorway. She might as well have asked, "Can you explain what kind of gambling is legal on Facebook?" My commute has rendered me more than a beat behind.

Before I can assess the contents of the refrigerator, the ceiling fan in the dining room diverts my attention. Every rotation further diminishes my concentration. On my way to turning it off, I spot the piles of clutter my roommate, a.k.a. my ex-husband, has left on the dining room table. Another assault on my ability to concentrate.

I reach into the fridge and emerge with a serving of some motley stew that has been stored in a round glass container, which can be taken on the road if dining in the car proves necessary. I have learned that it is better not to answer the loaded dinner question but rather to let my daughter reach peak hunger and then simply present something edible. I double or triple meals when I cook to ensure that there are always leftovers available.

My son recently left for college, but by sophomore year of high school, he was cooking dinner for himself most nights.

By the time my daughter has eaten her stew, it's time for the eight-mile street drive to my daughter's gymnastics practice, which is far mellower than my commute. While she tackles homework during the drive, I decompress in the quiet and daydream about my soothing hot bath only a few hours away.

The day I discovered a lavender bubble bath at the 99 Cents Only store, I felt as if I had won the lottery. Most perfume and candle scents irritate me, but the scent of lavender does the opposite. It calms me while I picture lavender fields in Provence.

CHAPTER 57

Career U-Turn

2018

After so many reorgs I lost count, my commute to Irvine finally ended July 27, 2018. My position had been eliminated along with most of my division's marketing team. I was terrified of relapsing. Since Bellevue, my only two relapses into mania had occurred during periods of unemployment. In 1993, it had actually been a period of underemployment as I had been working as a temp.

Because of all the reorgs, I had known that I might get laid off. In 2015, after the second reorg in less than a year, I had done some soul searching and gone back to school to supplement my elementary school teaching credential so I could teach high school. My high school teachers had fostered my love of learning, and I wanted to do the same.

It took a year to earn the high school credential. I had looked for a high school teaching job the past two summers and continued to do that in 2018. Because of skyrocketing rents and other factors, enrollments in some parts of Southern California had actually been dropping.

The insecurity during the job hunt brought me down. I had not felt like such crap for so long in years. I read something somewhere about learning to be comfortable with discomfort, and I told myself I could live with the pain. That I should say, *Thank you*, for feeling the pain, because that meant I was not numbing it.

One afternoon, when I took a break from my job search to research depression and anxiety symptoms for a freelance mental health article, I burst into laughter when I realized that what I was experiencing registered as anxiety and not depression.

So, this is why I used to take Ativan...

Financial insecurity and fear of homelessness have plagued me since childhood. Eight to ten hours a day, I was hunting for jobs in the three careers I have had, working with a job coach (courtesy of my former employer), and following companies on LinkedIn, yet I felt incredibly insecure. I was acting fine, but the pain in my chest was growing every day, until finally one day, I had to let go.

It's easy to have faith when things are going well, but the whole point of connecting with your spirit is to let go of ego and trust your higher power, the Universe, God, or whatever is more powerful than you. I let go of, *What if I don't find a job and can't support my children*, and the anxiety eased from on and off throughout the day to here and there throughout the week.

Something I had recently heard at a meeting helped too. A fellow recovering addict had shared, "I simply have to accept my chronic pain. It comes and goes, but it does go away for a while." It occurred to me that mild depression and anxiety were akin to chronic pain and that they did go away most of the time. Somehow, viewing it as chronic, intermittent pain helped me to be less afraid of it.

As far as not being able to find a job teaching, I realized that I would need to accept that if it was not meant to be. I had spent the last year volunteering with teens as a writing mentor and teaching career exploration skills at a continuation school, and there was no reason I could not continue to volunteer.

By September, the phone was starting to ring. I would answer the phone as my father had trained me to answer it, "Good afternoon. This is Sasha." When I was 12, part of becoming my father's social secretary had been to learn to answer the phone with a crisp, clear voice and to identify myself. This was probably to assure whatever woman that was calling that it was not another girlfriend answering the phone but his daughter.

One afternoon, I answered the phone and it was a recruiter calling. She had a professional sounding voice. A good sign. The job was a long-term temporary assignment working in something related to communications, and it paid well.

She described the various duties, which were similar to the job from which I had been laid off.

"Where is the job?"

"Downtown LA," she responded.

My heart thudded, but I cheerily responded, "It sounds like a great opportunity. Downtown L.A. was not what I had in mind, but I think it could work if I took the train."

"Great. I am going to send you the job description. If you want to tailor your resume a little bit, get back to me by tomorrow, and then I will submit your resume. It will probably take a week or so to hear anything back."

I thanked her, hung up the phone, and then immediately began researching my commuting options to Downtown LA. If parking was not covered by the employer, it could range from $200 a month to much more. Downtown LA was less than 30 miles from where I lived, but traffic began at 5 a.m. and was beyond unpredictable.

The commuter trains went through their bouts of unpredictability too, but I figured I could ride my bike the six miles each way to the train station two days a week and knock off two cardio workouts. It would take 20 minutes to drive the six miles to the station without traffic, because of a number of intersections. The days I drove to the train, it would take me one and a half hours each way to commute. The days I biked, it would take closer to two hours each way, but I would have gotten exercise out of the way.

Commuting is my worst stressor and challenges my mental health. It throws off my natural sleep cycle by forcing me to get up so early in the morning. I am not a night owl, but I am an evening owl. I cannot get to sleep before 10 p.m. no matter what. My natural time to get to sleep is 11 to 11:30 p.m. Having to get up at 5:20 a.m. to commute keeps me from working out in the morning. I hate the unpredictability of a nasty commute, and it makes it impossible to get to the doctor or any type of appointment during business hours.

Driving during rush hour is unnerving. But so is going into debt.

However, my son was in college and my daughter only had three years of high school left, so I knew I could move eventually. My daughter was thriving in our school district, which provided her with many varied opportunities. Her sports, clubs, and classes provided her with kind friends and committed, effective teachers. I would be loath to uproot her.

The economy was strong, and I landed a contract position teaching high school English within three months of having been laid off. The high school was near an off-ramp two exits before Los Angeles International Airport (LAX), which translated into 3 miles per hour traffic alongside travelers on the way to one of the busiest airports in the United States.

Without traffic, it took twenty-five minutes to travel the 19.6 miles from my home to the high school where I taught for two years until the summer of 2020. However, unless I left at 5 a.m., my morning commute took 45-50 minutes. The commute home took 60 to 70 minutes most days but could take up to 90 minutes or more. I listened to music, NPR, or podcasts to help ease the discomfort.

There are books and apps with checklists to help manage depression and bipolar disorder, but I run the below checklist in my head. My manias always came out of severe depression, so it became critical for me to monitor my depression. I often battle mild depression, but when it is mild, I can fight it and become free of it for hours, days, and even weeks.

Symptoms of mild depression

- Tightness in chest, whenever not engaged with a task
- Forcing myself to do tasks or anything
- Negative thoughts creeping in
- *What if?* beginning to dominate my thoughts

Am I moving beyond mild depression?

- Am I sleeping?
- Do I have an appetite?
- Am I able to concentrate and get work done?

- Am I showing up to appointments?

Some essential healthy habits

- Awareness of circadian rhythms and necessary accommodations

- Establish routines and structure

- Exercise five times (5X) a week

- Keep a gratitude journal

- Keep hydrated

- Maintain steady blood sugar

- Sleep at least seven (7) hours a night

- Spend at least 30 minutes outdoors during daylight

- Meditate (I am not as consistent with this one as I should be.)

CHAPTER 58

Benefits of Keeping a Gratitude Journal

While enjoying a sunset with my daughter at Sunset Beach, I noticed sunlight reflecting on the waves. The rays of sunlight slowly morphed into a golden ladder. At such times, a tiny jolt passes through me and the background fades away as I experience gratitude and freeze the moment in my thoughts.

During those moments, I feel completely relaxed. Later when I reflect on that moment, I reexperience the relaxation and gratitude.

One of my sponsors told me to begin a gratitude journal many years ago.

At times, I write my list on a scrap of paper. Generally, I write my list in a journal between dinner and bedtime. Sometimes, at bedtime, I am exhausted. If I haven't yet written my list,

I'm afraid to turn on the light lest it diminishes my sleepiness and makes it harder for me to get to sleep, and I recite my list in my head or write it down the next morning.

In May 2020, after eight months of a 70-hour-a-week workload, my teaching contract six weeks away from ending in the middle of a pandemic, and close to 20% unemployment in Los Angeles County, I was not feeling relaxed most of the time.

During stressful times, it seems that habits such as keeping a gratitude journal are most important. My chest is tight, I am crying on the inside, but I am functioning and even experiencing bits of joy and laughter that I can savor because I keep a gratitude journal.

Gratitude Journal Benefits

1. Shifts my focus from uncertainty and worries to whatever brought me joy that day.

2. Changes my thinking. After a few months of journaling, my thoughts during the day often go to, *I am so grateful for this. I want to put it on my list.*

3. Can be comforting before going to sleep or in the morning.

May 3, 2020

1. I got up early enough to say good-bye to my son who was headed back to college.

2. Read the Sunday *Los Angeles Times* on and off all day and got a feel for how other counties in California are experiencing COVID-19.

3. Two walks with the dog. Remembered to prompt him to sit before crossing the street (some of the time).

4. Dinner and watching *60 Minutes* together with the neighbors who have become extended family.

5. Got out a lengthy job application.

6. Four minutes of blow-drying my hair saved me from grabbing the kitchen scissors to cut my own eight months-since-a-haircut-hair. It made its flyaway texture bearable.

Find out more:

- "5 Reasons Keeping a Gratitude Journal Will Change Your Life," August 1, 2017, Goodnet.org.

- "5 Scientific Facts That Prove Gratitude is Good for You," November 28, 2013, Goodnet.org.

- Y. Joel Wong et al., "Does gratitude writing improve the mental health of psychotherapy clients? Evidence from a randomized controlled trial," March 28, 2018, *Psychotherapy Research*, 192-202.

CHAPTER 59

Meditation Helps You Manage Stress

Meditating can help change the way you manage the stress and anxiety that can lead to depression. Study after study has demonstrated that regularly meditating can rewire your brain.

Train your brain to focus

Stress and anxiety often lead to negative thinking and emotions, which can spiral out of control and immobilize you.

Meditation trains the brain to be able to sustain focus and to return to focusing on the task at hand instead of letting the negative thoughts and emotions take over.

Meditation rewires the brain

Regularly meditating can break the connection between the medial prefrontal cortex and the amygdala. The medial prefrontal cortex is the area of the brain in which you worry and ruminate. The amygdala produces the fight-or-flight response and triggers the release of the stress hormone cortisol. These two regions of the brain can interact to cause depression.

How does this work?

Meditation trains you to live in the present moment by teaching you how to focus on one thing at a time. When you experience the present moment—connect to your surroundings, feel alive, feel grounded—your mind lets go of negative thoughts.

You can't rewire your brain overnight. According to research, it takes at least eight weeks of daily meditation for changes in brain chemistry to occur, but you will notice smaller changes within days.

Many ways to meditate

There are many ways to meditate, but all you need to begin is a focal point, a simple constant. It could be:

- One word or a group of words repeated over and over
- A brief prayer, or part of a prayer
- A poem, or part of a poem
- Your breathing
- Your steps as you walk
- An object

You won't be able to instantly focus on one thing. Don't be discouraged. Even those who have practiced meditation for years struggle with wandering thoughts.

The process of attempting to achieve such focus is what rewires your brain and teaches you how to relax into the present moment.

Five minutes a day

Try it and keep trying it. Even five minutes a day helps. Five minutes a day almost every single day is more beneficial than longer sessions two or three times a week.

Schedule a daily time to meditate such as upon waking up. Once you start meditating you can fall into a looser state of meditation while walking or doing repetitive tasks like gardening.

At times of stress, you can slip into your routine meditation for a few seconds instead of immediately reacting.

Basic Meditation Exercise

This exercise typically doesn't work for me, but it is an easy, basic meditation that works for others.

1. Find a quiet place.

2. Close your eyes.

3. Choose a word for your focal point. Choose any word that comforts you when you repeat it.

4. Say your focus word silently to yourself each time you exhale.

5. When your mind wanders, gently return to your word or phrase.

6. Continue for five minutes. Gradually build up to ten or twenty minutes, if possible.

7. After meditating, sit quietly with your eyes closed for another minute or so before opening your eyes.

Seeing Meditation

Instead of a word, you can make an object your focal point.

1. Choose an object. Zoom in on it. Take several deep breaths as you sharpen your focus. Pretend that the object is the only thing that exists.

2. Try not to think about the object. Try not to have any thoughts at all. Try to simply see.

3. When thoughts arise, note them and return your focus to the object.

For fun, experiment with different types of objects.

- Stationary objects–such as a statue, a plant, or a chair

- Objects found in nature–such as the ocean, a tree, clouds, etc.

- Moving objects–such as a crowd, cars on a busy street, etc.

Stretch-Dance Meditation

For two years, I did this meditation for five to ten minutes a day. I have never felt so relaxed. I noticed that I lost track of time in a good way. I would wash the dishes and move on rather than constantly checking my watch to see if I would be done on time to take care of the next chore.

1. Pick a song that you adore. (I usually play the song from my phone.)

2. Play the song.

3. Feel the music. Absorb its rhythm.

4. Let the music guide you into stretching or dancing or a little bit of both.

5. Keep listening, stretching, dancing, or both until the end of the song.

6. Repeat the song and movement if necessary.

Some of my favorite songs lately for this exercise are "Drift Away" sung by Dobie Gray, "I Took a Pill in Ibiza" (Seeb Remix) by Mike Posner, "Airplanes" by B.o.B, "Payphone" by Maroon 5, "Thunder" by Imagine Dragons, and "Pompeii" by Bastille.

Find out more:

- Britta Hölzel et al. "Mindfulness practice leads to increases in regional brain gray matter density," *Psychiatry Research: Neuroimaging*, Volume 1919, Issue 1, January 30, 2011, p. 36-43, Harvard.edu.

- "How meditation helps with depression: A regular practice can help your brain better manage stress and anxiety that can trigger depression," *Harvard Health*, August 2018, Harvard.edu.

CHAPTER 60

How Do You Return to the Present Moment?

What if? can cascade into envisioning one catastrophe after another—each more terrifying than the one before.

I need tools to keep, *What if?* from escalating into incapacitating anxiety or depression. Usually, I use breathing exercises or take a break and do something physical, such as housework or yardwork. Here are some more tips.

1. Focus on your five senses, such as… Listen to the sounds around you. Feel the fabric of your clothes and focus on how they feel.

2. Look around as if you are seeing your surroundings for the first time.

3. Cultivate unselfconsciousness. Let go and stop thinking about your performance.

4. Focus on your breath. Allow mindfulness to make you more peaceful and smooth your interactions with others.

5. Enhance your engagement. Work on reducing moments of mindlessness and noticing new things to improve your mindfulness.

Find out more:

- "8 Ways to Return to the Present Moment" by Henrik Edberg, Updated March 23, 2020, PositivityBlog.com.

- "How to Live in the Present Moment: 35 Exercises and Tools (+ Quotes)" by Courtney E. Ackerman, MSc, April 26, 2020, PositivePsychology.com.

- "The Art of Now: Six Steps to Living in the Moment" by Jay Dixit, November 1, 2008, *Psychology Today*.

Epilogue

December 2020

It would have made quite a difference if, upon diagnosis, I had been taught about the role circadian rhythms and exercise play in bipolar depression. The skills I eventually learned, such as practicing gratitude, goal setting, and countering negative self-talk, enabled me to design a lifestyle that promotes my health and helps me manage my bipolar depression and addiction.

By learning new skills, the brain creates beneficial neural pathways within the nervous system. Once a new skill or skills are learned, applying these new skills strengthens those pathways. Healthy habits, such as exercise and eating whole foods can diminish the impact of harmful genes and increase the impact of beneficial genes. Some individuals are far more sensitive to their environments than others and environmental factors can also influence the impact of various genes.

I still struggle with depression and anxiety, but they don't take me down. I would be toast without regular exercise. It flips a switch for me like nothing else ever has, and it helps me sleep more soundly. Sleep = Balance = Stability.

As I write this, I occasionally experience tightness in my chest courtesy of anxiety due to the COVID-19 economy. I practice all my healthy habits and use the tools I have learned through step work and therapy, and I'm able to stay clean, show up, and to function *close* to my best. Gratitude reflections throughout the day do pierce through the anxiety.

Learning how to "act as if" helps. Acting as if means not waiting until I feel 100 percent to take care of a chore, sign up for a class, set up a meeting, or any other responsibility or challenge but just going ahead and taking the action anyhow. I can act my way out of feeling lousy, but waiting until I feel like taking the action could mean that I never take the necessary action and end up feeling even lousier.

Understanding the dynamics of the shaky circadian rhythms that tend to go along with bipolar disorder and how certain habits, especially those that disrupt sleep, can trigger episodes motivated me to establish routines. Interpersonal Social Rhythm Therapy (IPSRT) teaches individuals how to understand and work with their biological and social rhythms.

In addition to the spiritual aspect, recovery from active addiction took redesigning my lifestyle and rewiring some circuits in my brain so as to not constantly crave using. Brainstorming potential solutions rather than fixating on the problems is one part of the process.

Anxiety and ever-so-mild-depression that is far from clinical depression, but feels so, so awful, can trigger a relapse. I had to accept that my daily habits could contribute to that awful feeling and learn how to adjust them in order to make relapse unlikely.

Through the years, research has revealed much more regarding how to treat and manage mental health conditions, but there is less access to treatment. According to the Centers for Disease Control (CDC) September 11, 2020 "National Vital

Statistics Report," the national suicide rate for individuals aged 10-24 increased 57.4 percent between 2007 and 2018. Income inequality, racial injustice, and environmental injustice contribute to the significant gaps in access to healthcare.

I am haunted by the random circumstances that led me to effective wraparound treatment and that so many never end up receiving it.

Wraparound treatment could include follow-up outpatient care, health insurance, vocational counseling, training, supervised housing (if necessary), and health and lifestyle coaching. Although it is more involved at first, it is cost-effective because it can create productive members of society and reduce the need for recurrent critical care.

Let's stop divorcing mental health from brain health, addiction, trauma, and additional factors that could play a role in mental health, such as processing challenges, physical health, poverty, and discrimination. Let's take an integrative approach that addresses body, mind, spirit, social factors, and root causes and keeps manageable mental health conditions from escalating unnecessarily.

Taming bipolar

Accept it

Make peace with it

Do whatever it takes

Design your life to accommodate it

Sleep

Glossary

Adverse Childhood Experiences (ACES): From 1995 to 1997, Kaiser Permanente conducted the original ACE Study by collecting confidential surveys from over 17,000 of their San Diego HMO members regarding both their childhood experiences and their current health and circumstances profile. Similar studies through the years have replicated the results of the original ACE Study.

Ten of the most common types of childhood trauma are identified in the survey. Statistically, there tend to be negative consequences for those who have experienced four or more types of childhood trauma according to ACESTooHigh.com "Got Your ACE Score" section (https://acestoohigh.com/got-your-ace-score), "As your ACE score increases, so does the risk of disease, social and emotional problems. With an ACE score of 4 or more, things start getting serious. The likelihood of chronic pulmonary lung disease increases 390 percent; hepatitis, 240 percent; depression 460 percent; attempted suicide, 1,220 percent."

The "How Big is The problem?" subsection of the "Preventing Adverse Childhood Experiences" section of The Centers for Disease Control and Prevention's website (https://www.cdc.gov/violenceprevention/aces/fastfact.html) states, "About 61% of adults surveyed across 25 states reported that they had experienced at least one type of ACE, and nearly 1 in 6 reported they had experienced four or more types of ACEs."

"What are the consequences?" subsection of CDC.gov's "Preventing Adverse Childhood Experiences" section (https://www.cdc.gov/violenceprevention/aces/fastfact.html) offers further explanation:

> ACEs can have lasting, negative effects on health, well-being, and opportunity. These experiences can increase the risks of injury, sexually transmitted infections, maternal and child health problems, teen pregnancy, involvement in sex trafficking, and a wide range of chronic diseases and leading causes of death such as cancer, diabetes, heart disease, and suicide.
>
> ACEs and associated conditions, such as living in under-resourced or racially segregated neighborhoods, frequently moving, and experiencing food insecurity, can cause toxic stress (extended or prolonged stress).
>
> Toxic stress from ACEs can change brain development and affect such things as attention, decision-making, learning, and response to stress.

Children growing up with toxic stress may have difficulty forming healthy and stable relationships. They may also have unstable work histories as adults and struggle with finances, jobs, and depression throughout life. These effects can also be passed on to their own children. Some children may face further exposure to toxic stress from historical and ongoing traumas due to systemic racism or the impacts of poverty resulting from limited educational and economic opportunities.

Bipolar disorder (a.k.a. bipolar, bipolar depression, and manic depression):
The National Institute of Mental Health's website breaks down the different bipolar disorder diagnoses in its "Bipolar Disorder, Overview" section (https://www.nimh.nih.gov/health/topics/bipolar-disorder/index.shtml):

Bipolar disorder is a mental disorder that causes unusual shifts in mood, energy, activity levels, concentration, and the ability to carry out day-to-day tasks.

- Bipolar I Disorder—defined by manic episodes that last at least 7 days, or by manic symptoms that are so severe that the person needs immediate hospital care. Usually, depressive episodes occur as well, typically lasting at least 2 weeks. Episodes of depression with mixed features (having depressive symptoms and manic symptoms at the same time) are also possible.

- Bipolar II Disorder—defined by a pattern of depressive episodes and hypomanic episodes, but not the full-blown manic episodes that are typical of Bipolar I Disorder.

- Cyclothymic Disorder (also called Cyclothymia)—defined by periods of hypomanic symptoms as well as periods of depressive symptoms lasting for at least 2 years (1 year in children and adolescents). However, the symptoms do not meet the diagnostic requirements for a hypomanic episode and a depressive episode.

Sometimes a person might experience symptoms of bipolar disorder that do not match the three categories listed above, which is referred to as "other specified and unspecified bipolar and related disorders."

Circadian rhythm: Circadian rhythm is the 24-hour internal clock controlled by the hypothalamus (a region of the forebrain) that affects hormonal cycles, body temperature, and your sleep/wake cycle. Ideally, your circadian rhythm should cycle between sleepiness and alertness at regular intervals throughout the day.

Cognitive Behavioral Therapy (CBT): CBT is a type of talk therapy that aims to change thought patterns and perceptions by identifying negative, harmful thoughts, challenging them, and finding alternative, more constructive, ways to deal with those thoughts.

Psychiatrist Aaron Beck founded CBT in the 1960s. It also has roots in Rational Emotive Behavioral Therapy (REBT), which was founded by psychologist Albert Ellis.

Collective unconscious: The unconscious refers to that part of the mind containing memories and impulses of which you're not aware. Psychiatrist Carl Jung came up with the concept of the collective unconscious in 1916 to identify the part of the deepest unconscious that is derived from ancestral memory and experience, genetically inherited, common to all humankind, and separate from the part of the unconscious shaped by the individual's personal experience.

Cyclothymia: Individuals diagnosed with cyclothymia experience low-grade depression and mild symptoms of hypomania.

Depression: Depression can occur as a reaction to loss or tragedy. Depression is characterized by a sense of hopelessness, difficulty concentrating, loss of interest in everyday activities, loss of energy, difficulty sleeping or sleeping too much, and loss of appetite or overeating. Clinical depression can occur without any triggering event and is depression that lasts all day, every day, for two weeks or more and can include recurring thoughts of death or suicide.

Dialectical Behavioral Therapy (DBT): DBT is a type of cognitive behavioral therapy that generally uses individual weekly psychotherapy sessions in conjunction with weekly group therapy sessions. It is often used to treat suicidal and other self-destructive behaviors.

The individual sessions focus on problem-solving behavior strategies and how they are being used on a daily basis. The weekly group therapy sessions teach skills from four different modules: interpersonal effectiveness, distress tolerance/reality acceptance, emotion regulation, and mindfulness.

Epigenetics: Epigenetics is the study of biological processes that affect which genes are expressed, switched on. The processes do not modify the DNA sequence of the genes, but instead, they affect how cells "read" the genes, whether or not the genes are expressed.

Lifestyle and environment influence gene expression. Ideally, we would aim to suppress the expression of harmful genes and promote the expression of beneficial genes.

"A Super Brief and Basic Explanation of Epigenetics for Total Beginners," September 1, 2019, WhatIsEpigenetics.com, https://www.whatisepigenetics.com/what-is-epigenetics/.

Rachael Rettner, "Epigenetics: Definition & Examples," June 24, 2013, LiveScience.com, https://www.livescience.com/37703-epigenetics.html.

Genetics: Genetics is the study of genes, heredity, and the variation of inherited characteristics.

Hypomania: Hypomania, by definition, does not cause impairment or psychosis, a break from reality. According to "Ask the doctor: What is hypomania?" published on the Harvard Health website, hypomania would be diagnosed when at least three of the following symptoms persisted for at least four days: grandiosity, decreased need for sleep, increased talkativeness, racing thoughts, noticeable distractibility, agitation or increased activity, and risky behavior, such as overspending, impulsive business investments, and promiscuity.

For mania to be diagnosed, the article states, "… symptoms are mostly the same, except they last at least one week, lead to hospitalization, or include psychotic symptoms (a break with reality)."

"Ask the doctor: What is hypomania," Harvard Health Publishing, Updated June 19, 2019, https://www.health.harvard.edu/staying-healthy/what-is-hypomania.

Inflammation: Your body's white blood cells and what they produce use the process of Inflammation to protect you from harmful invaders, such as bacteria and viruses. Chronic, long-lasting, inflammation is linked to a number of diseases, such as heart disease, cancer, and depression.

Overconsumption of sugar has been linked to chronic inflammation. In addition to desserts, sugar is added to most processed foods to improve flavor and increase shelf life.

"The Sweet Danger of Sugar," November 5, 2019, Harvard Health Publishing, Health.Harvard.edu, https://www.health.harvard.edu/heart-health/the-sweet-danger-of-sugar.

Interpersonal and Social Rhythm Therapy (IPSRT): IPSRT teaches individuals with mood disorders how to improve their moods and prevent episodes by understanding and working with their biological and social rhythms. (Find out more at IPSRT.org.)

Mania: Decreased need for sleep, increased energy, elation, euphoria, unpredictability, bouts of irritability, impulsivity, recklessness, and impaired judgment characterize mania. Mania can be diagnosed if symptoms last most of the day, nearly every day, for at least one week.

Mindfulness: When you entirely focus your awareness on the present moment, you experience mindfulness.

Mixed Episode: During a mixed episode, individuals experience high and low symptoms, mania and depression, at the same time.

Neuroimaging: Neuroimaging, a.k.a. brain imaging, is the process of directly or indirectly producing images of the structure, function, or pharmacology of the brain or other parts of the nervous system. Neuroimaging techniques include magnetic resonance imaging (MRI) or computerized tomography.

PTSD (Post-Traumatic Stress Disorder): PTSD is a long-term debilitating reaction that can occur when someone experiences or witnesses a traumatic event or series of events. Symptoms can include unpredictable emotions, flashbacks, nightmares, strained relationships, headaches, and nausea.

"What is Posttraumatic Stress Disorder?" American Psychiatric Association, Psychiatry.org, https://www.psychiatry.org/patients-families/ptsd/what-is-ptsd.

Subconscious: The subconscious is the part of the mind below the conscious level. It involves memories, beliefs, fears, and subjective interpretations of reality. Although you are not aware of your subconscious mind, it influences your actions and feelings.

Trauma: Living through or witnessing a deeply distressing event, or events, causes psychological or emotional trauma. Brain scans have revealed that trauma changes the structure and function of the brain and may impair the ability to function after the traumatic event or events have occurred.

APPENDIX B

Discussion Points

Part 1: Trauma

1. Describe any childhood events that you consider traumatic.

2. How did you deal with those events as a child and as a teen?

3. Calculate your ACE (Adverse Childhood Experiences) score and help place it in context by visiting https://www.npr.org/sections/health-shots/2015/03/02/387007941/take-the-ace-quiz-and-learn-what-it-does-and-doesnt-mean.

4. Learn even more by checking out the CDC ACE Study website https://www.cdc.gov/violenceprevention/aces/. How is an ACE score significant in relation to mental health conditions?

5. While growing up, do you feel as if some of the adults in your life lived in denial?

Part 2: Chaos

1. Describe any times as a teen or young adult in which you acted out?

2. What tricks do you use to help you focus?

3. Describe the times in your life that your creativity became more of a curse than a blessing.

4. Why is it so important to have someone truly listen to you? To be heard? What happens when you aren't?

Part 3: Awareness

1. Bellevue Hospital offered wraparound treatment and outpatient follow-up. Why do you think this makes a difference?

2. How would you define addiction?

3. Describe the circumstances in which you or anyone you know traded addictions?

4. How do certain addictions differ in their impact? How are they similar?

5. Why do you think Sarah was so influential as a therapist? How was she influential?

Part 4: Awakening

1. How can becoming a parent shift your perspective? Inspire you? Create additional stressors? Affect your career?

2. What are some of the additional challenges a newborn can present to someone with bipolar disorder?

3. What strategies did the author use to be able to sleep in spurts while her son slept so that she could fight off hypomania?

4. How could a processing challenge influence mental health? If you or anyone close to you has wittingly or unwittingly struggled with a processing challenge, such as ADD or dyslexia, describe the impact.

5. What are the traits that go along with sugar sensitivity? How can sugar sensitivity become sugar addiction? What are the consequences of sugar addiction?

6. How might feelings intensify when you let go of sugar addiction?

7. Give examples of how step work can help you change your thinking patterns to more constructive ones.

8. Describe the highly sensitive trait. What are some ways a highly sensitive individual could accommodate it? How could it interfere with depression, anxiety, or bipolar disorder?

9. Describe the temperaments of a dandelion, a tulip, and an orchid. Which one are you?

Part 5: Insight

1. What role do you think shame plays in managing mental health conditions? How does American culture promote shame when it comes to mental health conditions?

2. Name some obvious and some less obvious triggers for depression or mania.

3. Describe the ways in which commuting can be stressful.

4. How can seeking approval become a negative influence?

5. In what ways can the dynamics of group therapy be more effective than individual therapy?

6. How can a checklist help you maintain your mental health? What items would you put on your own checklist?

7. What benefits do meditation, keeping a gratitude journal, returning to the present moment, and humor offer?

8. How can you use any of these methods to fight stress or depression?

APPENDIX C

Notes

INTRODUCTION: The Web

Judith Lewis Herman, *Trauma and Recovery: The Aftermath of Violence – From Domestic Abuse to Political Terror* (Basic Books, 2015)

NOTE TO READER

National Alliance on Mental Illness, NAMI In Our Own Voice, https://www.nami.org/Support-Education/Mental-Health-Education/NAMI-In-Our-Own-Voice.

Shorter, Edward, "DSM-5 Will be the last," May 14, 2013, Oxford University Press blog, https://blog.oup.com/2013/05/dsm-5-will-be-the-last/.

CHAPTER 5: Circadian Rhythms and Bipolar Depression

Yoshikazu Takaesu, "Circadian rhythm in bipolar disorder: A review of the literature," *Psychiatry and Clinical Neurosciences.* 2018 Sep:72(9) p. 673-682, https://pubmed.ncbi.nlm.nih.gov/29869403/.

CHAPTER 9: Overmedicated

Moodswing: The Third Revolution in Psychiatry, Ronald Fieve, MD, (Morrow, 1975), *Moodswing: Dr. Fieve: The Eminent Psychiatrist Who Pioneered the Use of Lithium in America Reveals a Revolutionary Way to Fight Depression* (Second Revised Edition, Penguin Random House, 1989)

A. Coppen et al., "Decreasing lithium dosage reduces morbidity and side-effects during prophylaxis," Volume 5, Issue 4, November 1983, *Journal of Affective Disorders*, p. 353-362, https://www.sciencedirect.com/science/article/abs/pii/0165032783900265.

"Lithium Treatment Over the Lifespan in Bipolar Disorders," May 7, 2020, *Frontiers in Psychiatry*, https://www.frontiersin.org/articles/10.3389/fpsyt.2020.00377/full.

CHAPTER 11: Q&A Interview With Dr. Laryssa Creswell: Long-Term Effects of Childhood Trauma

Laryssa M. Creswell, Ed.D., MT-BC, LPC, LCPC Operations Manager/Therapist-Empowered Connections, LLC, Adjunct Professor, The Chicago School of Professional Psychology, Washington DC, via email September 30, 2020.

Judith Lewis Herman, MD, *Trauma and Recovery: The Aftermath of Violence—From Domestic Abuse to Political Terror* (Basic Books, 2015)

Laura S. Brown, Mary Ballou, *Rethinking Mental Health & Disorder: Feminist Perspectives* (The Guilford Press, 2002)

CHAPTER 12: Nineteen

John Bradshaw, *Bradshaw On the Family: A New Way of Creating Solid Self-Esteem* (Health Communications Inc., 1996)

CHAPTER 15: NA Meeting

Narcotics Anonymous (NA), Narcotics Anonymous World Services, https://www.na.org/.

CHAPTER 20: ADHD, ADD, and Creativity

Holly White, "The Creativity of ADHD: More insights on a positive side of a disorder,'" March 5, 2019, *Scientific American*, https://www.scientificamerican.com/article/the-creativity-of-adhd/.

Eunice N.Simões et al., "What does handedness reveal about ADHD? An analysis based on CPT performance," June 2017, *Research in Developmental Disabilities* p. 45-56, https://www.sciencedirect.com/science/article/abs/pii/S0891422217301063.

CHAPTER 21: How Can Setting Goals Help

You Focus?

Zawn Villines, "Effective Goal Setting Could Help People with Depression," January 5, 2017, GoodTherapy.org, https://www.goodtherapy.org/blog/effective-goal-setting-could-help-people-with-depression-0105171.

Leslie Riopel MSc., "The Importance, Benefits, and Value of Goal Setting," April 26, 2020, PositivePsychology.com, https://positivepsychology.com/benefits-goal-setting/.

CHAPTER 24: Sleeping With the Enemy

Alex Berenson, *Tell Your Children: The Truth About Marijuana, Mental Illness, and Violence,* (Simon and Schuster, 2019)

CHAPTER 32: Q&A Interview With Dr. Roger McIntyre: Bipolar Depression and "Addiction"—The Relationship

Roger McIntyre, PhD, Professor of Psychiatry and Pharmacology, University of Toronto, Director of Depression and Bipolar Support Alliance (DBSA), via email June 26, 2020.

CHAPTER 33: Routines Benefit Depression and Bipolar Depression

Sasha Kildare, "Routine Maintenance: How Sticking to a Schedule Helps Maintain Balance," *bp Magazine*, Winter 2017, https://www.bphope.com/routine-schedule-maintain-balance-bipolar/.

Interpersonal and Social Rhythm Therapy, ipsrt.org, https://www.ipsrt.org/.

Mariana Plata, MSc, "The Power of Routines in Your Mental Health," October 4, 2018, *Psychology Today.com*, https://www.psychologytoday.com/us/blog/the-gen-y-psy/201810/the-power-routines-in-your-mental-health.

Brain and Behavior Research Foundation, "Circadian Rhythms and Bipolar Disorder," April 9, 2019, BBRFoundation.org, https://www.bbrfoundation.org/event/circadian-rhythms-and-bipolar-disorder.

CHAPTER 34: Anxiety, Depression, and Low Self-Compassion—The Relationship

Kristen Neff, "Why Self-Compassions Trumps Self-Esteem," May 27, 2011, *Greater Good Magazine*, https://greatergood.berkeley.edu/article/item/try_selfcompassion.

Amy Louise Finlay-Jones, "The relevance of self-compassion as an intervention target in mood and anxiety disorders: A narrative review based on an emotion regulation framework," *Clinical Psychologist* 21 (2017) 90–103.

Nicole Snaith et al., "Mindfulness, self-compassion, anxiety and depression measures in South Australian yoga participants: implications for designing a yoga intervention," *Complementary Therapies in Clinical Practice*, Volume 32, August 2018: 92-99, https://pubmed.ncbi.nlm.nih.gov/30057066/.

Alexander C Wilson. et al., "Effectiveness of Self-Compassion Related Therapies: a Systematic Review and Meta-analysis," *Mindfulness* (2019) 10:979–995, https://link.springer.com/article/10.1007/s12671-018-1037-6.

CHAPTER 36: Postpartum

Overeaters Anonymous (OA), https://oa.org/.

CHAPTER 38: Sugar Sensitivity

Fern Reiss, *The Infertility Diet: Get Pregnant and Prevent Miscarriage*, (Peanut Butter and Jelly Press, 1999)

"Radiant Recovery" website addressing sugar addiction, https://radiantrecovery.com/.

CHAPTER 42: Sylvia

The Power of Now: A Guide to Spiritual Enlightenment by Eckhart Tolle (Namaste Publishing, 1999).

Cocaine Anonymous (CA), Cocaine Anonymous World Services, ca.org.

CHAPTER 43: On Stage

Don Miguel Ruiz, *The Four Agreements: A Practical Guide to Personal Freedom (A Toltec Wisdom Book)*, (Amber-Allen Publishing, 1997).

Erma Bombeck Writer's Workshop, University of Dayton, Ohio, https://udayton.edu/artssciences/initiatives/erma/.

CHAPTER 45: Will Effective Treatment for Addiction Ever Become the Norm?

Sasha Kildare, "Will effective treatment for addiction ever become the norm," October 6, 2016, DrivenToTellStories.com, https://driventotellstories.com/will-effective-treatment-for-addiction-ever-become-the-norm/2016/sashakildare/.

Gabrielle Glaser, "The Irrationality of AA," April 2015, *The Atlantic*.

Adam Finberg, *The Business of Recovery*, March 27, 2015, Greg Horvath Productions, https://www.thebusinessofrecovery.com/.

Richard A. Friedman MD, "Taking Aim at 12-Step Programs," May 5, 2014, *The New York Times*, https://www.nytimes.com/2014/05/06/health/the-sober-truth-seeing-bad-science-in-rehab.html.

Lance Dodes, MD and Zachary Dodes, *The Sober Truth: Debunking the Bad Science Behind 12-Step Programs and the Rehab Industry*, (Beacon Press, 2014).

James Clear, *Atomic Habits: An Easy & Proven Way to Build Good Habits & Break Bad Ones*, (Penguin Books, 2018).

Sarah A. Benton MS, LMHC, LPC, AADC, "Irrationality of AA? A critique of the recent *Atlantic* article," March 25, 2015, PsychologyToday.com, https://www.psychologytoday.com/us/blog/the-high-functioning-alcoholic/201503/irrationality-aa.

Katie MacBride, "The Irrationality of *The Atlantic's* piece on AA," April 3, 2015, Addiction.com. https://www.addiction.com/blogs/the-irrationality-of-the-atlantics-piece-on-aa/.

Joseph Nowinski, PhD, *If You Work It, It Works!: The Science Behind 12-Step Recovery*, (Hazelden, 2015).

Tommy Rosen, "Spirituality vs. Science? A Rebuttal to *The Atlantic* Article, 'The Irrationality of Alcoholics Anonymous,'" March 20, 2015, *Huffington Post*, https://www.huffpost.com/entry/spirituality-versus-scien_b_6909290.

Jesse Singal, "Why Alcoholics Anonymous Works," March 17, 2015, TheCut.com, https://www.thecut.com/2015/03/why-alcoholics-anonymous-works.html.

CHAPTER 46: Interview with Dr. Ted Zeff: Are You Highly Sensitive?

Ted Zeff, PhD author of *The Power of Sensitivity: Success Stories by Highly Sensitive People Thriving in a Non-sensitive World*, (phone interview, August 28, 2017).

CHAPTER 47: Temperament, Trauma, and Sensitivity

Vincent J Felitti MD, FACP, et al., "Relationship of Childhood Abuse and Household Dysfunction to Many of the Leading Causes of Death in Adults: The Adverse Childhood Experiences Study (ACE) Study," *American Journal of Preventive Medicine*, May 1, 1998, Volume 14, Issue 4: 245-258, https://www.ajpmonline.org/article/S0749-3797(98)00017-8/fulltext.

Nadine Burke Harris, MD, MPH, California Surgeon General, "How Childhood Trauma Affects Health Across a Lifetime," TEDMED 2014, September 2014, https://www.ted.com/talks/nadine_burke_harris_how_childhood_trauma_affects_health_across_a_lifetime?language=en.

Francesca Lionetti, Arthur Aron, Elaine N Aron, et al., "Dandelions, tulips and orchids: evidence for the existence of low-sensitive, medium-sensitive and high-sensitive individuals," *Translational Psychiatry*, January 22, 2018, https://doi.org/10.1038/s41398-017-0090-6.

David M. Greenberg et al., "Elevated empathy in adults following childhood trauma," PLoS ONE, 3(10): e0203886,

October 3, 2018, https://journals.plos.org/plosone/article/related?id=10.1371/journal.pone.0203886.

Zachary Wallmark et al., "Neurophysiological effects of trait empathy in music listening," April 6, 2018, https://www.frontiersin.org/articles/10.3389/fnbeh.2018.00066/full.

CHAPTER 51: Addicted to Approval

"Bipolar Disorder/Symptoms and Causes," MayoClinic.org, https://www.mayoclinic.org/diseases-conditions/bipolar-disorder/symptoms-causes/syc-20355955.

CHAPTER 52: Group Therapy for Codependency

Independent Writers of Southern California (IWOSC), http://www.iwosc.org.

CHAPTER 53: Mr. Smooth

Sasha Kildare, "L.A. Affairs: How she plans to manifest Mr. Right and get off the dating merry-go-round for good," September 5, 2015, *Los Angeles Times*, https://www.latimes.com/home/la-hm-affairs-20150905-story.html.

California Council on Problem Gambling, calpg.org.

Lisa Jones et al., "Gambling problems in bipolar disorder in the UK: prevalence and distribution," October 2015, p.328-333, *The British Journal of Psychiatry*, https://www.cambridge.org/core/journals/the-british-journal-of-psychiatry/article/gambling-problems-in-bipolar-disorder-in-the-uk-prevalence-and-distribution/FFDC24125902367FCC0EDACB05E025B9.

CHAPTER 58: Benefits From Keeping a Gratitude Journal

"5 Reasons Keeping a Gratitude Journal Will Change Your Life," August 1, 2017, Goodnet.org, https://www.goodnet.org/articles/5-reasons-keeping-gratitude-journal-will-change-your-life.

"5 Scientific Facts That Prove Gratitude is Good for You," November 28, 2013, Goodnet.org, https://www.goodnet.org/articles/5-scientific-facts-that-prove-gratitude-good-for-you.

Y. Joel Wong et al., "Does gratitude writing improve the mental health of psychotherapy clients? Evidence from a randomized controlled trial," March 1, 2018, *Psychotherapy Research*, Volume 28(2):192-202, https://www.tandfonline.com/doi/abs/10.1080/10503307.2016.1169332?src=recsys-&journalCode=tpsr20.

CHAPTER 59: Meditation Helps You Manage Stress

Britta K. Hölzel et al., "Mindfulness practice leads to increases in regional brain gray matter density," January 30, 2011, *Psychiatry Research: Neuroimaging*, Volume 191(1):36-43. https://pubmed.ncbi.nlm.nih.gov/21071182/.

"How meditation helps with depression: A regular practice can help your brain better manage stress and anxiety that can trigger depression," August 2018, *Harvard Health Publishing*, https://www.health.harvard.edu/mind-and-mood/how-meditation-helps-with-depression.

CHAPTER 60: How Do You Return to the Present Moment?

Henrik Edberg, "8 Ways to Return to the Present Moment," Updated March 23, 2020, PositivityBlog.com, https://www.positivityblog.com/8-ways-to-return-to-the-present-moment/.

Courtney E. Ackerman, MSc, "How to Live in the Present Moment: 35 Exercises and Tools (+ Quotes)," January 9, 2020, PositivePsychology.com, https://positivepsychology.com/present-moment/.

Jay Dixit, "The Art of Now: Six Steps to Living in the Moment," November 1, 2008, *Psychology Today*, https://www.psychologytoday.com/us/articles/200811/the-art-now-six-steps-living-in-the-moment.

APPENDIX D

Recommended Reading

1. *All the Things We Never Knew, Chasing the Chaos of Mental Illness* by Sheila Hamilton (Seal Press, 2015). Sheila Hamilton's former husband and the father of their child committed suicide weeks after receiving his diagnosis of bipolar disorder. This compelling memoir and information guide seeks to answer why.

2. *Atomic Habits: An Easy & Proven Way to Build Good Habits & Break Bad Ones* by James Clear (Penguin Books, 2018). *Atomic Habits* explains how cue, craving, response, and reward influence nearly every action we take, how to systematically create beneficial habits, how to get rid of detrimental habits, and much more. Highly engaging.

3. *The Bell Jar (25ᵗʰ Anniversary Edition)* by Sylvia Plath (Harper Collins, 1996). The most exacting description

I have ever read of a gradual descent into psychotic depression. Darkly humorous at times, *The Bell Jar* also gives the reader a window into the constraints faced by women in the 1950s.

4. *Bradshaw On the Family: A New Way of Creating Solid Self-Esteem* by John Bradshaw (Health Communications inc., 1996). Bradshaw explains the dynamics surrounding addiction, including the compulsivity that fuels addiction and how compulsivity can lead to trading addictions.

5. *Driven to Distraction: Recognizing and Coping with Attention Deficit Disorder from Childhood through Adulthood* by Edward M. Hallowell, MD and John J. Ratey, MD (Simon & Schuster, 1994).

6. *Just Like Someone Without Mental Illness Only More* by Mark Vonnegut (Bantam, 2011). During the same year Vonnegut was named Boston Magazine's "No. 1 Pediatrician," he ended up hospitalized with his fourth psychotic break following years of self-medication with alcohol and prescription pills.

7. *Lost Marbles: Insight Into My Life With Bipolar and Depression* by Natasha Tracy (Natasha Tracy, 2016). Tracy's book shares her own experience with bipolar disorder as well as advice for others who have been diagnosed with it and advice for their loved ones.

8. *Are We Failing Our Kids? Mental Health and Education* by Andrea Shaker (New Degree Press, 2021)

9. *Strung Out: One Last Hit and Other Lies That Nearly Killed Me* by Erin Kahr (Park Roe, 2020) More than a memoir, *Strung Out* examines the psyche and culture driving the addiction.

For Real Health Ed and Career Ed

For insight into why our education system is failing our neediest students and what is needed to improve it, check out "The State of American Education" 1A WAMU NPR broadcast/podcast.

Three tweaks to today's educational system could help teenagers when it comes to addressing addiction or managing mental health conditions.

- Motivate more students by teaching them about career options beginning in middle school, including the ability to pursue a trade at 16.

- Integrate health (including mental health) education into the science curriculum throughout middle school and high school.

- Make the learning process more of a hands-on experience.

Professions include trades

America is lending money it doesn't have to kids who can't pay it back to train them for jobs that no longer exist. That's nuts." – Mike Rowe

Former *Dirty Jobs* host Mike Rowe's quote sums it up. He created a foundation that gives scholarships for skilled trades job training.

Teens and young adults who are on their own today are extremely vulnerable. It is nearly impossible now to get a job straight out of high school in which you can support yourself. If you can't support yourself, where do you live? How do you eat?

We end up tacitly shaming many American youths who aren't inclined toward academics but have other talents that they do not get a chance to discover because they get turned off by what is offered to them.

We should be telling teenagers… You can be the best you can be, but it takes work to figure out your strengths and likes.

For the most part, our high school system is set up to prepare students for an academic path through college and possibly graduate school. We should be preparing students to have the option to pursue a trade at 16, not 18. It is no longer feasible to set up trade programs, such as auto mechanics, ultrasound or x-ray technology, and culinary, at high schools but those programs can be found at nearby community colleges.

- It's too expensive to feed and clothe a teen for two more years (from 18 to 20), if not necessary.

- Beginning in middle school, students should have career education in their curriculum so that they can develop an eye for careers, begin exploring the options their community colleges provide, begin assessing their own strengths and affinities, and learn research and interviewing skills.

- Between 16 and 18, many disengaged students begin routinely abusing drugs and/or fall into depression. By 18, most of these students no longer have the motivation, confidence, or organizational skills to figure out and pursue a trade at a community college.

- If a teen truly hates school and can't relate to the academic curriculum, they become far more alienated by 18.

- Many disengaged 16-year-olds would buy in to education if they knew it led to a job that paid real money and provided independence (the option to move out of the house).

Health and mental health education

Health and mental health concepts, such as nutrition, the importance of sleep, routines, movement, exercise, and more should be integrated into the science curriculum throughout junior high and high school.

Rethinking the learning experience

The learning experience should be made more active, more practical, more relatable and incorporate more project-based learning.

Christopher Emdin's book *For White Folks Who Teach in the Hood... and the Rest of Y'all Too: Reality Pedagogy and Urban Education* offers case studies, research, insight, and potential solutions to the disconnect for less affluent youth in our public education system.

Find out more:

- Mike Rowe Works Foundation, https://www.mikeroweworks.org/.

- *For White Folks Who Teach in the Hood... and the Rest of Y'all Too: Reality Pedagogy and Urban Education* by Christopher Emdin (Beacon Press, 2016)

- 1A: The State of American Education, WAMU, National Public Radio (NPR), December 17, 2019, https://the1a.org/segments/2019-12-17-the-state-of-american-education/ (Guests: Alejandro Gibes de Gac, CEO & Founder Springboard Collaborative; Amanda Ripley, author, *The Smartest Kids in the World: And How They Got That Way*; Natalie Wexler, education journalist, author, *The Knowledge Gap: The Hidden Cause of America's Broken Education System—and How to Fix It*; and Andreas Schleicher, Director for Education and Skills, Organization for Economic Co-operation and Development.)

Mental Health and Addiction Resources

Below are some established national organizations and a few Southern California ones. Online, find local and regional organizations by typing keywords into a search engine, such as mental health peer support groups, warmline directory, county department of mental health + your county, and addiction support groups.

National Suicide Prevention Hotline
24 hrs / 7 days: 1-800-273- TALK (8255)
Crisis Text Line: Text "START" to 741-741+

SAMHSA Disaster Distress Helpline
24 hrs / 7 days: 1-800-985-5990
Crisis Text Line: Text "TalkWithUs" to 66746
TTY: 1-800-846-8517

2-1-1 Information and Referral Line
Call 2-1-1 for help with food, housing, employment, health care, counseling, and more.
211.org

Find a Treatment Facility
FindTreatment.gov (Find a treatment facility near you.)

12-Step Organizations
This lists most 12-step organizations. Their respective websites provide meeting directories, schedules of events, and links to resources.

Al-Anon Family Groups, al-anon.org
Alcoholics Anonymous (AA), aa.org
Co-Dependents Anonymous (CODA), coda.org
Debtors Anonymous (DA), da.org
Gam-Anon, gam-anon.org
Gamblers Anonymous (GA), gamblersanonymous.org
Narcotics Anonymous (NA), na.org
Overeaters Anonymous (OA), oa.org
Sex and Love Addicts Anonymous (SLAA), slaafws.org

Depression and Bipolar Alliance (DBSA)
dbsalliance.org
800-826-3632

DBSA is a nationwide grassroots network that provides peer-based, wellness-oriented support, education, and services online and through local support groups for individuals with mood disorders.

LA County Department of Mental Health
dmh.lacounty.gov
24 / 7 Help Line: 800-854-7771
Crisis Text Line: Text "LA" to 741741

There are county mental health departments throughout the US. LA County Department of Mental Health is an example of one. Mental health services provided include assessments, case management, crisis intervention, medication support, peer support, and other rehabilitative services.

Mental Health America
mhanational.org

Community-based non-profit aiming to address the needs of those living with mental illness by providing education, outreach, information, referral services, research, innovation, policy, and advocacy.

NAMI, National Alliance for Mental Illness
nami.org
Main: 703-524-7600
Member Services: 888-999-6264
Information Hotline: 800-950-NAMI (6264)

NAMI's Top 25 HelpLine Resources: nami.org/Support-Education/NAMI-HelpLine/Top-HelpLine-Resources

NAMI, an alliance of more than 600 local affiliates, provides advocacy, education, support, and public awareness to enable individuals and families affected by mental illness to build better lives.

National Institute of Mental Health (NIMH)
nimh.nih.gov
nimh.nih.gov/health/index.shtml (Mental Health Information)
866-615-6464

NIMH is the lead federal agency for mental health research. The Mental Health Information page on its website links to information, research, and topics related to mental health.

Project Return: Peer Support Network

prpsn.org
323.346.0960
Warmline English: 888.448.9777 (A warmline is a peer-run listening line.)
Warmline Spanish: 888.448.4055

Project Return Peer Support Network offers a variety of services ranging from self-help groups, support hotlines, a respite house for individuals in the midst of a crisis, resource centers, career and employment support, and training and consultation to other organizations. It is based in Southern California, but there are similar organizations in other parts of the country.

Recovery International

recoveryinternational.org
312-337-5661
866-221-0302

"The mission of Recovery International is to use the cognitive-behavioral, peer-to-peer, self-help training system developed by Abraham Low, MD, to help individuals gain skills to lead more peaceful and productive lives."

RI International

riinternational.org
866-481-5361
Local and TTY/TDD: 602-650-1212

RI International's services include crisis, outpatient, housing, community support teams, and more. They have more than 50 programs located throughout the United States and abroad.

SAMHSA, Substance Abuse and Mental Health Services Administration

samhsa.gov
FindTreatment.gov (Find a treatment facility near you.)

SAMHSA's National Helpline:
800-662-HELP (4357)
TTY: 800-487-4889

SAMHSA is the agency within the U.S. Department of Health and Human Services tasked with reducing the impact of substance abuse and mental illness on communities throughout the US.

SAMHSA's 24-hour National Helpline provides free and confidential referrals and information regarding mental and/or substance use disorders, prevention, treatment, and recovery in English and Spanish.

With Hope

withhopefoundation.org
714-524-1996

"With Hope, the Amber Craig Memorial Foundation is a non-profit organization dedicated to suicide prevention through improving mental health awareness and education in our schools and throughout our community."

How Can Movement Help Zap Depression?

There are many activities that help fight depression and anxiety. Over the years, I've relied on exercise and moving around to help me relax, concentrate, and sleep more soundly.

In addition to exercise, there are many surprisingly simple ways to move around. I've summarized and illustrated some of the most practical ways in a bonus chapter.

You can download the "Move" chapter at:
DrivenToTellStories.com/Move

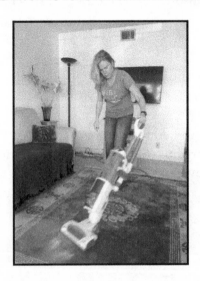

Nuances of Storytelling and the Link Between Creativity and Depression

Inspiration—often from surprising sources—can captivate you. Storytelling enables you to express yourself, inspire others, and connect to the community as well as other creatives.

Once or twice a month, I blog about the art, craft, and business of storytelling in its many forms and the relationship between creativity and depression.

Subscribe to the blog at:
DrivenToTellStories.com

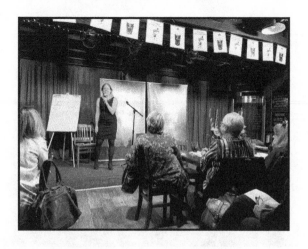

Watch a Klutzy Middle-Aged Mom Demonstrate Quick Tips on Fighting Depression and Anxiety

Beginning weekly in April 2021, I will upload 1- to 2-minute videos featuring tips on how to fight mild to moderate depression and anxiety. As I clumsily demonstrate them, I will briefly explain the science behind these tips.

Subscribe: YouTube Sasha Kildare

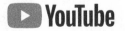

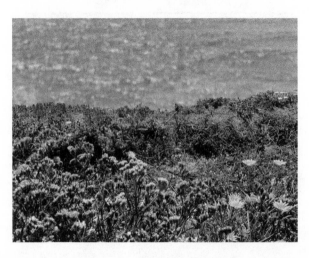

9 781647 466633